Upper-Extremity Task-Specific Training After Stroke or Disability: A Manual for Occupational Therapy and Physical Therapy

**Catherine E. Lang, PhD, PT, and
Rebecca L. Birkenmeier, OTD, OTR/L**

With Contributions From
Marghuretta D. Bland, DPT, MSCI, PT, NCS, and
Jill M. Seelbach, DPT, PT

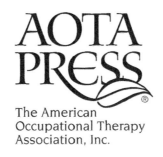

AOTA PRESS

The American
Occupational Therapy
Association, Inc.

AOTA Centennial Vision

We envision that occupational therapy is a powerful, widely recognized, science-driven, and evidence-based profession with a globally connected and diverse workforce meeting society's occupational needs.

Mission Statement

The American Occupational Therapy Association advances the quality, availability, use, and support of occupational therapy through standard-setting, advocacy, education, and research on behalf of its members and the public.

AOTA Staff

Frederick P. Somers, *Executive Director*
Christopher M. Bluhm, *Chief Operating Officer*

Chris Davis, *Director, AOTA Press*
Ashley Hofmann, *Development/Production Editor*
Jennifer Folden, *Marketing Specialist*
Amanda Fogle, *Marketing Specialist*

American Occupational Therapy Association, Inc.
4720 Montgomery Lane
Bethesda, MD 20814
Phone: 301–652–AOTA (2682)
TDD: 800–377–8555
Fax: 301–652–7711
www.aota.org
To order: 1–877–404–AOTA or store.aota.org

Disclaimers

This publication is designed to provided accurate and authoritative information in regard to the subject matter covered. It is sold or distributed with the understanding that the publisher is not engaged in rendering legal, accounting, or other professional service. If legal advice or other expert assistance is required, the services of a competent professional person should be sought.
—*From the Declaration of Principles jointly adopted by the American Bar Association and a Committee of Publishers and Associations*

It is the objective of the American Occupational Therapy Association to be a forum for free expression and interchange of ideas. The opinions expressed by the contributors to this work are their own and not necessarily those of the American Occupational Therapy Association.

ISBN: 978-1-56900-349-7

Library of Congress Control Number: 2013951868

Cover Design by Debra Naylor, Naylor Design, Inc., Washington, DC
Composition by Maryland Composition, Laurel, MD
Printed by Automated Graphic Systems, Inc., White Plains, MD

Acknowledgments

We are grateful for the contributions of Eliza M. Prager, OTD, MSCI, OTR/L; Kimberly J. Waddell, MS, OTR/L; and Emily S. Grattan, MS, OTR/L, to the task development process. Thanks to Brittany Hill for her assistance with editing.

Contents

About the Authors and Contributors

Authors

Catherine E. Lang, PhD, PT

Dr. Lang is Associate Professor in the Program in Physical Therapy, Program in Occupational Therapy, and Department of Neurology at Washington University in St. Louis. She received her physical therapy degree from the University of Vermont in 1993 and her doctorate in movement science from Washington University in 2001. She completed a postdoctoral fellowship at the University of Rochester between 2001 and 2004.

The long-term goal of Dr. Lang's research studies program is effective and efficient individualized neurorehabilitation. Her primary study population is people with stroke, and the majority of her research studies examine movement and the upper extremity. Research efforts include characterizing neurobehavioral changes over the course of stroke recovery, developing new and optimizing current motor interventions, and improving clinical practice. Work in the laboratory is supported by the National Institutes of Health, the American Heart Association, and various private foundations.

Rebecca L. Birkenmeier, OTD, OTR/L

Dr. Birkenmeier is Research Assistant Professor in the Program in Occupational Therapy, Program in Physical Therapy, and Department of Neurology at Washington University in St. Louis. She graduated from Truman State University with a bachelor's degree in psychology in 1998 and earned her master's degree in occupational therapy from Washington University School of Medicine in 2001. She went on to receive her occupational therapy doctorate from Washington University School of Medicine in 2010.

Dr. Birkenmeier currently works in the Neurorehabilitation Research Lab at Washington University School of Medicine with Dr. Lang. She provides the occupational therapy perspective for several of the lab's ongoing research studies and was responsible for developing the task-specific training protocol with Dr. Lang.

Contributors

Marghuretta D. Bland, DPT, MSCI, PT, NCS

Dr. Bland is a Board-Certified Neurologic Clinical Specialist and an Assistant Professor of Physical Therapy, Neurology, and Occupational Therapy at Washington University School of Medicine. She received her doctor of physical therapy from Washington University in 2008 with a master's degree in clinical investigation.

Her clinical experience includes inpatient rehabilitation for people with spinal cord injury, outpatient services for people with stroke, and general acute care. In addition to her other academic responsibilities, Dr. Bland currently serves as the Coordinator for the Brain Recovery Core Project, a collaboration between Washington University, Barnes Jewish Hospital, and The Rehabilitation Institute of St. Louis to improve care and outcomes for people who have had a stroke.

Jill M. Seelbach, DPT, PT

Dr. Seelbach earned her doctor of physical therapy degree in 2010 from the Washington University in St. Louis Program in Physical Therapy. She spent time working at the Rehabilitation Institute of Chicago, where her clinical focus was on stroke and brain injury.

Dr. Seelbach currently works as a Research Physical Therapist under the mentorship of Dr. Lang in the Neurorehabilitation Research Laboratory at Washington University in St. Louis.

List of Figures, Tables, Exhibits, and Case Examples

Introduction

Catherine E. Lang, PhD, PT, and Rebecca L. Birkenmeier, OTD, OTR/L

Upper-Extremity Task-Specific Training After Stroke or Disability: A Manual for Occupational Therapy and Physical Therapy draws on decades of clinical research and practice. Although current evidence strongly supports task-specific training for upper-extremity (UE) rehabilitation, there was a need for a resource consolidating research and providing practical, useful information on how to apply task-specific training in clinical practice.

When we and others publish research articles, restrictions on the number of words limit the amount of detail that can be provided in a methods section. Published articles can be frustrating when information is insufficient for readers to understand exactly what was done and how the intervention was delivered. Without key details, it can be difficult to deliver task-specific training, especially when trying to tailor training to the individual needs of a client. This manual was designed to fill that information gap.

What Is Task-Specific Training?

Task-specific training involves the active, repetitive practice of functional activities to learn or relearn a motor skill. Other terms that are often used interchangeably with task-specific training include *task-oriented training* and *repetitive task practice*. Although these alternate terms may have slightly different meanings across professional disciplines or research groups, these terms represent the same conceptual idea of repeated, challenging practice of functional, goal-oriented activities.

Task-specific training has emerged as an efficacious intervention, whether used by itself or in combination with other interventions (e.g., constraint-induced movement therapy, functional electric stimulation). Most clinicians would agree that the goal of rehabilita-tion is to help an individual gain (or regain) the capacity to complete important functions for daily life. Task-specific training, as usually portrayed in the literature, can be used for restoring or remediating UE motor control. However, it is important to note that task-specific training can also be used in a compensatory manner for facilitating recovery of functional abilities.

This manual is written from the perspective of our research in persons with stroke, but task-specific training can be applied to persons with other neurological conditions and even for persons with nonneurological conditions (e.g., surgery, trauma) who have the goal of improving functional use of the UE. Similarly, although the manual addresses UE task-specific training, its general ideas and principles could easily be expanded to other body parts or actions that are goals of rehabilitation treatment.

How This Manual Is Organized

The manual is logically arranged such that the order of the chapters mirrors the demands of clinical practice. Chapter 1, "Overview of Task-Specific Train-ing," introduces task-specific training, describes why it is an emerging choice for treatment, provides a general overview of task-specific training principles, and discusses the unique challenges of UE task-specific training.

Chapter 2, "Assessment for Task-Specific Train-ing," includes information on assessing sensorimotor impairments and UE function activity and identifying and setting goals. Chapter 3, "Task-Specific Training," contains information needed to individualize and implement task-specific training, including goal setting, task selection, and task set-up.

Chapter 4, "Toolbox of Upper-Extremity Tasks," contains 100 tasks, including self-care, productivity, and leisure tasks. Chapter 5, "Planning and Organizing Tasks Into a Treatment Program," provides general guidelines for how to organize tasks into a treatment program. Chapter 6, "Task-Specific Training as the Home Exercise Program," describes how to use this training as a home program.

It is anticipated that users of this manual may read each chapter once and then use Chapter 4, "Toolbox of Upper-Extremity Tasks," on a daily basis as they provide rehabilitation services.

The exciting part of task-specific training is that it nourishes the creativity of clinicians. It takes some good detective work to match the goals, interests, and motor capabilities of a client to specific, challenging motor tasks for them to practice. We find that we are always generating new, interesting ideas for tasks and hope you will, too.

CHAPTER 1
Overview of Task-Specific Training

How to Use This Manual

The purposes of this book are to (1) introduce students and clinicians to task-specific training and the science that underlies it and (2) provide a how-to manual that can be used to implement task-specific training in daily rehabilitation service delivery.

This manual is intended for occupational therapists, physical therapists, and therapy assistants using task-specific training with their clients. Although the manual focuses on task-specific training for people with stroke, task-specific training can be used with people with other neurological conditions (e.g., traumatic brain injury, spinal cord injury) and even with people with nonneurological conditions (e.g., surgery, trauma) who have the goal of improving functional use of the upper extremity (UE). Similarly, although the manual addresses UE task-specific training, the general ideas and principles could easily be expanded to other body parts or actions that are goals of rehabilitation treatment.

The manual provides a general overview of task-specific training for the UE. Later chapters contain the information needed to individualize and implement task-specific training, including assessments, goal setting, task selection, and task set-up. Chapter 4, "Toolbox of Upper-Extremity Tasks," and the longest chapter, contains 100 tasks for practitioners to use with their clients. The final chapters provide general guidelines on how to organize tasks into a treatment program and how to use this training as a home program. Because the intent of task-specific training is to help a person gain (or regain) the capacity to complete functional tasks, clinicians will find that task-specific training will be beneficial for most of their clients.

Task-specific training can be used on its own or in combination with other interventions, and it can be applied with the goal of acquiring compensatory function or of restoring previously lost function. We antici-

pate that users of this manual may read each chapter once and then use Chapter 4, "Toolbox of Upper-Extremity Tasks," on a daily basis as they provide rehabilitation services.

Introduction to Task-Specific Training

Task-specific training involves the active, repetitive practice of functional activities in an effort to learn or relearn a motor skill (Bayona, Bitensky, Salter, & Teasell, 2005; Hubbard, Parsons, Neilson, & Carey, 2009). Time spent repeatedly practicing tying one's shoes is a common clinical example of task-specific training for someone who wants to be independent in self-care activities. It is intuitive that practicing a skill can result in improved performance of that skill, which is true for general motor skills, such as hitting a baseball, and rehabilitation skills, such as bathing, grooming, and writing. No one would expect time spent catching a baseball to result in improved performance in hitting a baseball. Similarly, one should not expect practicing single-joint exercises (e.g., elbow flexion and extension) to result in improved reaching performance or grasping a therapy cone to result in improved grooming skills.

Task-specific implies that the person is participating in behavioral experiences that directly replicate the sensorimotor demands that need to be acted on to execute the motor skill successfully. In other words, the person is engaging in a functional activity that has been identified as a rehabilitation goal. *Training* implies that the behavioral experiences are not just repetition of the same thing but involve ongoing challenge to a person's capabilities. Just as a runner training for a marathon does not run the same distance at the same pace in each session, a person participating in rehabilitation would not repeatedly practice the same action in the same way and at the same level of difficulty in each session.

The idea of providing an ongoing, gradual challenge to learn a skill arose many decades ago in the field of psychology and is called *shaping* (Peterson, 2004). Shaping is a fundamental principle in the development of task-specific UE rehabilitation (Bayona et al., 2005; Hubbard et al., 2009; Krakauer, 2006; Teasell et al., 2008; Taub et al., 1993; Winstein et al., 2003; Woldag, Stupka, & Hummelsheim, 2010). Lately, research has shown that this need for ongoing challenge through shaping is a critical factor in improving functional outcomes (Taub et al., 2013).

Other terms that are often used interchangeably with *task-specific training* include *task-oriented training* and *repetitive task practice*. Although these alternate terms may have slightly different meanings across some professional disciplines or research groups, they represent the same conceptual idea of repeated, challenging practice of functional, goal-oriented activities.

Task-Specific Training as an Emerging Choice for Treatment

The neuroscience and rehabilitation literatures are converging to strongly support the idea that extended task-specific training is critical for producing lasting changes in motor system networks, motor learning, and motor function (Kleim, Barbay, & Nudo, 1998; Kleim & Jones, 2008; Kleim, Jones, & Schallert, 2003; Plautz, Milliken, & Nudo, 2000; Shepherd, 2001; Teasell et al., 2008). People with stroke and other neurological conditions are benefiting from this emerging treatment choice (Bayona et al., 2005; Hubbard et al., 2009; Teasell et al., 2008).

Insights into the neural mechanisms of motor learning through task-specific training are largely derived from animal models of stroke recovery. Repeated training of challenging movements stimulates the molecular pathways of learning and memory within the motor system (Adkins, Boychuk, Remple, & Kleim, 2006). Training potentiates the specific neuronal connections that are used (called *long-term potentiation,* or *LTP*). The persistence of LTP resulting from training over days and weeks facilitates motor system connectivity through formation of new synapses *(synaptogenesis),* growth of new axonal branches *(axonal sprouting),* formation of new blood vessels *(angiogene-*

sis), and potentially generation of new neurons *(neurogenesis)* in animal models of stroke (Carmichael, 2008; Nudo, Plautz, & Frost, 2001).

These molecular and cellular changes manifest as enhanced motor cortical representations of the newly acquired movement. Enhanced cortical representations resulting from task-specific training have been clearly demonstrated in both human and animal studies (Hlustik & Mayer, 2006; Karni et al., 1995, 1998; Liepert, Graef, Uhde, Leidner, & Weiller, 2000; Nudo, 2006; Nudo & Milliken, 1996; Nudo, Milliken, Jenkins, & Merzenich, 1996; Pascual-Leone, Grafman, & Hallet, 1994). Indeed, thousands of repetitions of challenging motor tasks result in larger brain representations of the practiced movement (Adkins et al., 2006; Carey et al., 2002, 2004; Nudo, 2007; Nudo et al., 1996, 2001). Moreover, large amounts of task-specific training are the key part of efficacious UE rehabilitation interventions, such as constraint-induced movement therapy (Wolf et al., 2006).

Many trials have tested various methods of task-specific training, either alone or in combination with other interventions. For example, *constraint-induced movement therapy* is intensive task-specific training paired with restraint of the unaffected limb and a behavioral plan to facilitate transfer of therapy training to real-world activity (Taub, Uswatte, & Pidikiti, 1999). Likewise, task-specific training has been evaluated when paired with many other therapy options such as wrist orthoses (Barry, Ross, & Woehrle, 2012), electrical stimulation (Knutson et al., 2012), and brain stimulation (Stinear, Barber, Coxon, Fleming, & Byblow, 2008). Despite the difficulties in interpreting vastly different experimental designs in relatively small samples, the general consensus is that rehabilitation of the UE should involve task-specific training of functionally relevant activities (U.S. Department of Defense & U.S. Department of Veterans Affairs, 2010).

Principles of Task-Specific Training

To help guide the implementation of task-specific training, we have compiled a short list of principles.

- Practice of a movement results in improvement in that movement.

- Large amounts of practice are required to truly master a motor skill. The ideal dose of practice is unknown.
- Learning requires solving the motor problem, not rote repetition of overlearned tasks.
- Learning does not occur in the absence of feedback.
- Intrinsic feedback is optimal for promoting self-learning and generalization.
- Optimal learning occurs with high levels of motivation and engagement.
- Variable practice conditions are optimal for learning and generalization.
- Within-session, massed practice promotes learning better than within-session distributed practice.
- Practice of a whole task results in better learning than practice of parts of the task, unless the task can be broken down into clearly separable components.

Table 1.1 lists each principle, how the principle is implemented in animal studies and human motor learning studies, and how the principle might be used to structure task-specific training. This information is primarily derived from reviews and book chapters (Hubbard et al., 2009; Kleim & Jones, 2008; Winstein & Stewart, 2006).

In subsequent chapters of this book, we use these principles and provide additional information about how they are applied to task-specific UE training.

Challenges of Upper-Extremity Task-Specific Training

A major challenge of UE task-specific training is the enormous number of UE tasks that may need to be addressed. This training is different from task-specific training of the lower extremity, for which the list of tasks that need to be practiced may be relatively short, for example, transfers, walking, and stairs. As people move through daily life, they execute many tasks with the UEs. Even considering a single daily routine such as dressing, a person has to be able to don and doff undergarments, socks, pants, shirt, belt, watch, and so forth. If one multiplies the number of daily routines by the number of tasks within each routine, the result is a very large number of tasks in specific contexts that need to be performed daily by any given person.

A challenge related to UE task-specific training is the problem of generalization of training. Practice and improved performance of one task have largely been assumed to generalize, or transfer, to improved performance on other tasks, but limited data exist to support or refute this idea with respect to the motor skills that are the focus of rehabilitation. Numerous studies from the neuroscience literature have examined transfer of movement training in highly controlled laboratory tasks (e.g., Ghahramani & Wolpert, 1997; Goodbody & Wolpert, 1998; Shadmehr & Moussavi, 2000). The general conclusions derived from these and other similar studies are that transfer across tasks can occur, but it is relatively limited in scope. Newer studies of generalization on tasks that are a closer match to rehabilitation skills have suggested that practice of one task results in small improvements (10%) on other, nonpracticed tasks in healthy people (Schaefer & Lang, 2012) and in people with stroke (Schaefer, Patterson, & Lang, 2013).

To help address these challenges, it is useful to think about UE tasks on the basis of their component parts. Most UE movement tasks can be divided into four essential components: (1) reach, (2) grasp, (3) move or manipulate, and (4) release (Lang, 2012).

Distinctions between tasks are based on the order of the components and the specifics of each component, such as where to reach, which type of grasp to use, and how much force is needed (Lang, 2012). People undergoing rehabilitation may have difficulty with all four essential components or with only one or two in specific contexts. A systematic assessment of underlying impairments and functional actions will assist the therapist in determining which components should be the focus of practice (see Chapter 2, "Assessment for Task-Specific Training"). Practice of the components in specific contexts may then be matched to a client's interests and goals and appropriately graded to challenge the client's motor capabilities (see Chapter 3, "Task-Specific Training"). Because therapy services are limited, it is impossible to practice all tasks in rehabilitation. Thus, clinicians must choose wisely when determining which tasks to practice and how to prac-

Table 1.1. Principles to Guide Task-Specific Training

Principle	Insights and Implementation in Animal Models and Motor Learning Studies	Implementation in the Clinic
Practice of a movement results in improvement in that movement.	• Animals practice purposeful movements: reach–grasp–retrieve.	• Individual tasks incorporate the essential components of reach, grasp, move or manipulate, and release.
Large amounts of practice are required to truly master a motor skill. The ideal dose of practice is unknown.	• Animals perform hundreds of repetitions daily for up to 3 months. • Animal and human studies have not yet determined an optimal number of daily repetitions. • Brain reorganization continues for a short while after behavior plateaus.	• Large amounts of task-specific practice are needed, more than what is provided in routine care. • Practice outside of therapy sessions is strongly encouraged. • Consider ways to encourage practice even when therapy services have ended.
Learning requires solving the motor problem, not rote repetition of overlearned tasks.	• Brain reorganization occurs with learning, not simply with repetition.	• Tasks can be graded to increase difficulty. Progression to higher levels of difficulty continually challenges the client's motor capabilities.
Learning does not occur in the absence of feedback. Intrinsic feedback is optimal for promoting self-learning and generalization.	• Animals have clear intrinsic feedback on each trial about knowledge of results (i.e., eat the food pellet or not).	• Tasks have clear goals so clients can easily determine knowledge of results. • Clients can be given summary feedback on knowledge of results (number of repetitions achieved, number of successful completions, time spent) at the end of each task.
Optimal learning occurs with high levels of motivation and engagement.	• Animals are food deprived, and the task is to retrieve food, creating very high levels of motivation and engagement.	• Clients help to select tasks for practice to increase engagement and motivation. • Tasks can be changed, as needed, to minimize boredom. • Individual clients practice 2–4 tasks each session to minimize boredom.
Variable practice conditions are optimal for learning and generalization.	• Animals practice a single task under limited variable conditions (e.g., changing well sizes or well locations).	• Essential movement components stay the same, but the context of the components changes. • Variation is accomplished across tasks (e.g., practice of multiple tasks) and within tasks (e.g., by varying objects, location, weight, speed, accuracy).

(Continued)

Table 1.1. Principles to Guide Task-Specific Training *(Cont.)*

Principle	Insights and Implementation in Animal Models and Motor Learning Studies	Implementation in the Clinic
Within-session massed practice promotes learning better than within-session distributed practice.	• Animals continually perform their movement task throughout the session.	• The environment is set up to allow for continuous practice. • Individual clients are given encouragement by the practitioner to continue practicing. • Rest breaks are provided only at the client's request.
Practice of a whole task results in better learning than practice of parts of the task, unless the task can be broken down into clearly separable components.	• Animals practice the whole task of retrieving and eating a pellet.	• Basic underlying movement components of reach, grasp, move or manipulate, and release represent a whole sequence of movements as performed in the real world.

tice them (see Chapter 4, "Toolbox of Upper-Extremity Tasks"; Chapter 5, "Planning and Organizing Tasks Into a Treatment Program"; and Chapter 6, "Task-Specific Training as the Home Exercise Program").

Summary

In summary, task-specific training involves the repeated, challenging practice of functional, goal-oriented activities. Task-specific training is an intervention choice that is well supported in the literature for people with neurological conditions, particularly those with stroke. Principles derived from human and animal learning studies guide the implementation of task-specific training for people receiving UE rehabilitation services. Considering UE movements as a series of component movements (i.e., reach, grasp, move or manipulate, and release) can facilitate individualized task selection and generalization.

CHAPTER 2   Assessment for Task-Specific Training

Assessment of the upper extremity (UE) is necessary to determine the initial level of UE impairment, function, and activity. Assessment results are compared with a client's rehabilitation goals to determine whether the goals are achievable or they need to be adjusted. After goals are determined, assessment results guide selection of one or more interventions and are used to tailor the selected interventions to achieve the client's goals. In addition, results from UE function and activity measures serve as a baseline from which to document improvement or the absence of improvement during and after rehabilitation services. The intent of this chapter is to provide a method of assessment for implementing UE task-specific training; a comprehensive review of all UE assessments is beyond the scope of this manual.

Assessment of Sensorimotor Impairments

Delivery of effective, appropriate UE rehabilitation depends on selecting appropriate interventions and tailoring interventions to each client. Thus, each client receiving UE rehabilitation services should undergo an assessment that determines the presence and severity of sensorimotor impairments. In this section, we provide a brief conceptual overview of the four most common UE sensorimotor impairments: (1) paresis, (2) loss of fractionated movement, (3) abnormal tone, and (4) somatosensory loss (Sathian et al., 2011).

Another sensorimotor impairment, ataxia, is seen in about 5% of people with stroke.[1] *Ataxia* is a motor coordination deficit in which movements are inaccurate and highly variable. Two additional impairments highly relevant to UE rehabilitation are neglect and apraxia. *Neglect* is an attentional deficit resulting in altered perceptions and is the result of disruption of attentional brain networks. *Apraxia* is a collection of deficits in motor planning and is the result of disrup-

tion of frontal and parietal lobe motor planning networks. Task-specific training as described in this text is not an intervention that specifically targets ataxia, neglect, or apraxia per se. Nonetheless, considering their presence and severity when implementing task-specific training is useful. These impairments are important to consider because

- Task-specific training may be able to partially address these impairments;
- How task-specific training is implemented may need to be different when these impairments are present; and
- The presence and severity of these impairments may influence outcomes (see Chapter 5, "Planning and Organizing Tasks Into a Treatment Program," for specific modifications related to ataxia, neglect, and apraxia).

For a thorough description of all of these impairments and their underlying neural mechanisms, readers are referred to several published reviews (Buxbaum et al., 2004; Corbetta, Kincade, Lewis, Snyder, & Sapir, 2005; Lang, 2012; Lang, Bland, Bailey, Schaefer, & Birkenmeier, 2013; Petreska, Adriani, Blanke, & Billard, 2007; Sathian et al., 2011; Wheaton & Hallett, 2007).

Figure 2.1 provides a conceptual map linking damaged brain networks to the five most common sensorimotor impairments, impairments to their common clinical terms, and impairments to a few general assessment tools. Starting at the top of Figure 2.1, damage to the nervous system, such as from stroke, results in neuronal death. Disruption of nervous system functions occurs both at the site of the lesion and across the brain networks of which the lesioned site is a part (Carter, Shulman, & Corbetta, 2012). Structural and functional damage across each network results in the sensorimotor impairments of paresis, loss of fractionated movement, abnormal muscle tone, somatosen-

---

[1] Based on unpublished data from Washington University of ~15,000 patients.

Figure 2.1. Conceptual map linking damaged brain networks to impairments, impairments to common clinical terms, and impairments to brief assessment tools.

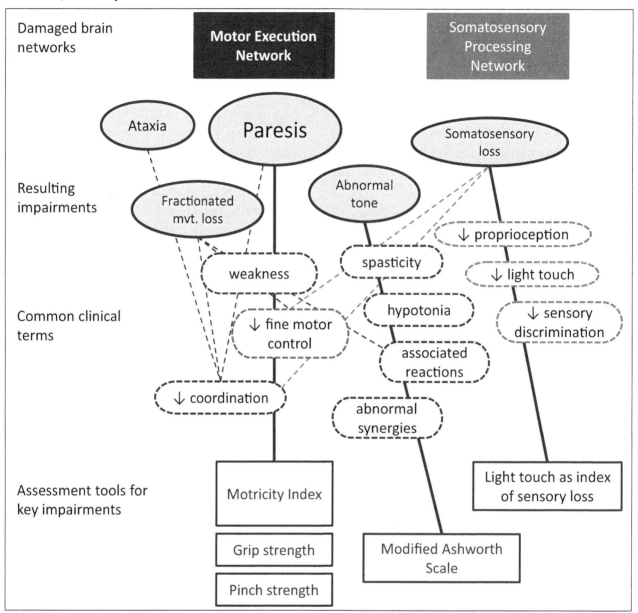

Note. Impairments stemming from motor and somatosensory networks are shown in the solid oval shapes. Dotted ovals indicate common clinical terms that reflect both motor and somatosensory impairments. Rectangles indicate assessment tools for key impairments. mvt. = movement.

sory loss, and ataxia (Sathian et al., 2011). *Paresis* is an inability to volitionally activate spinal motor neuron pools. The most common clinical terms for paresis are *weakness* and *decreased strength.*

Loss of fractionated movement is the inability to move a joint or segment by itself, for example, attempts to flex the elbow result in simultaneous flexion at the shoulder, wrist, and fingers. Common clinical terms describing loss of fractionated movement in-

clude synergistic movement and associated reactions. Muscle tone can be either too high (i.e., *hypertonicity*) or too low (i.e., *hypotonicity*). The most common clinical term for abnormal muscle tone is *spasticity.* Somatosensory loss after central nervous system damage generally affects multiple somatosensory modalities, such that people have decreased proprioception, light touch, and sensory discrimination abilities. Other common clinical terms, as seen in Figure 2.1, are the product of multiple impairments. For example, decreased fine motor control is due to paresis, loss of fractionated movement, and possibly somatosensory loss. Similarly, decreased coordination can be due to paresis, loss of fractionated movement, somatosensory loss, and ataxia.

Note that paresis is displayed prominently in Figure 2.1 because it is the primary contributor to poststroke loss of UE activity and function (Beebe & Lang, 2008, 2009a; Lang & Beebe, 2007; Prager & Lang, 2012), which makes sense intuitively because one needs to be able to activate motor neuron pools to move a UE segment. Without the ability to move or move well, UE function is clearly compromised.

The assessment tools shown along the bottom of Figure 2.1 measure key sensorimotor impairments; quantification of these impairments is needed to design an UE task-specific training program. Note that this list is not an exhaustive one of all possible ways to measure the impairments. The assessments are intended as a basic, minimal battery (for review, see Bland et al., 2013; Lang et al., 2013) from which task-specific training interventions can be individualized and implemented. Table 2.1 provides a description of each measure and additional details for ease of use in clinical practice.

Assessment of Upper-Extremity Function and Activity

Management of a client's care after stroke in a rehabilitation setting should focus not just on minimizing impairments but also on maximizing function (Duncan et al., 2005). When achieving improved function in daily activities is the goal of both the client and the clinician, performing assessments that evaluate UE function is imperative. Early standardized evaluations using functional assessments are a critical component of developing a comprehensive treatment plan (Duncan et al., 2005). Assessments of UE function are often omitted from the initial evaluations because they add time. Moreover, many rehabilitation facilities follow a formal assessment protocol that nearly exclusively measures at the level of impairment and the level of disability (assistance needed) but does not include a specific UE function measure. In this section, we pro-

vide examples of UE functional assessments, and in Chapter 3, "Task-Specific Training," we discuss how to use these assessments to create an individualized task-specific training program.

Many UE functional assessment measures are available. These assessments are highly interrelated and are often easy to administer (for a review, see Lang et al., 2013). Functional assessments can be divided into two categories: (1) performance measures in which the therapist rates or times a series of UE movements performed by the client and (2) self-report measures in which the therapist asks the client a series of questions about UE movements. Here, we present two functional assessment measures in both categories that are particularly useful for task-specific training (see Table 2.2 for additional details on each measure). Functional measures presented in this chapter are meant to be a guide for the development of task-specific training tasks found in this manual. We selected measures on the basis of established reliability and validity in stroke and other neurological patient populations (Connell & Tyson, 2012). Because most UE measures are highly interrelated, that is, they quantify the same underlying construct (Beebe & Lang, 2009b), there is flexibility in choosing a specific measure to use.

Performance Measures

Action Research Arm Test

The Action Research Arm Test (ARAT; Lyle, 1981) is a 19-item assessment designed to evaluate changes in UE function as a result of paresis. Clients handle a variety of objects on four subscales (Grasp, Grip, Pinch, and Gross Motor Movement) and are then rated on a scale ranging from 0 (*cannot perform desired movement*) to 3 (*performs the movement normally*). The ARAT is reliable and valid to use in the stroke population, takes roughly 10 to 15 minutes to administer, and can be purchased commercially or built from specifications reported in research studies (Lyle, 1981; Yozbatiran, Der-Yeghiaian, & Cramer, 2008).

Box and Block Test

The Box and Block Test (BBT; Mathiowetz, Volland, Kashman, & Weber, 1985) is a quick performance assessment that measures unilateral UE dexterity. Cli-

Table 2.1. Minimal Set of Assessments to Quantify the Presence and Severity of Upper-Extremity Sensorimotor Impairments, Particularly for Clients With Stroke

Impairment and Assessment	Description	Additional Notes	Time to Administer
Paresis			
MI (Collin & Wade, 1990; Demeurisse, Demol, & Robaye, 1980)	The MI is MMT for 3 UE movements: shoulder abduction, elbow flexion, and pinch grip. The 3 MMT scores are converted to a total force production score for each UE movement, ranging from 0 *(no strength)* to 100 *(full strength)*.	Paresis after stroke affects movement similarly at each UE segment, which means that one needs to test only a few UE segments, not all. The MI is a quick version of MMT and provides a total force score for the entire UE. Interrater reliability = .88	<5 minutes
Grip strength and pinch strength: Dynamometer (Mathiowetz, Kashman, et al., 1985; Mathiowetz, Weber, Volland, & Kashman, 1984)	A commercially available handheld dynamometer is used to quantify kilograms or pounds of grip or pinch force. Age- and gender-appropriate normative values are available.	Handgrip strength is a reliable predictor of motor performance and functional independence (Heller et al., 1987; Sunderland, Tinson, Bradley, & Hewer, 1989) Intrarater reliability = .80, interrater reliability = .97	3 minutes
Movement: Observation of fractionated movement during paresis assessment	Note the presence or absence of individuated movement at UE segments; watch for substitutions or associated reactions.	As part of the paresis assessment, fractionation of movement can be assessed.	No additional time
Tone: MAS (Bohannon & Smith, 1987a)	Resistance to passive movement at different speeds is quantified on a 6-point scale ranging from 0 *(no increase in muscle tone)* to 4 *(affected part is rigid)*.	The elbow flexors and finger flexors are most easily and commonly assessed in the UE. Tone at these segments will be similar to tone at other UE segments. Interrater reliability = .85	5 minutes
Light touch sensation: Light stroke	Light touch sensation is typically noted as intact, impaired (i.e., less feeling compared with other side), or absent on the basis of one light stroke to the skin of the UE.	Loss of somatosensation after stroke typically occurs across multiple modalities and across the entire limb. Light touch is the most easily assessed. If light touch is decreased at 1–2 representative sites, it is an indicator that similar deficits exist in other modalities (e.g., proprioception) and at other locations.	2 minutes

Note. MAS = Modified Ashworth Scale; MI = Motricity Index; MMT = manual muscle testing; UE = upper extremity.

ents are asked to pick up and move small 1-inch blocks over a divider one at a time. The number of blocks moved in 1 minute is recorded for both limbs. Scores are then compared with established norms. The BBT is reliable and valid for use in the stroke population, takes roughly 5 minutes to administer, and can be purchased commercially for a relatively low cost.

We selected both the ARAT and the BBT assessments because they are considered to be robust and clinically useful measures of UE function (Connell &

Table 2.2. Minimal Set of Functional Assessments to Quantify Upper-Extremity Function, Particularly for Clients With Stroke

Assessment	Other Considerations	Reliability	Concurrent Validity (r)	Time to Administer
Performance measures				
ARAT	Valid and reliable for all time points poststroke; allows observation of grasp and manipulation of multiple objects	Intrarater = .99 Interrater = .98 Test–retest = .98	r = .91–.94 with Fugl-Meyer Motor Assessment r = .96 with Motor Assessment Scale r = .87 with MI r = .93 with CAHAI	10–15 minutes
BBT	Quick to administer; allows observation of grasp of only one object; must have some degree of fine motor control to move a block	Intrarater = NA Interrater = .99 Test–retest = .96	r = .92 with Fugl-Meyer Motor Assessment r = .95 with ARAT	5 minutes
Self-report measures				
MAL	Tries to capture real-world abilities from many questions; subject to self-report biases	Test–retest = .79–.82	r = .35–.39 (QOM scale) with ARAT r = 0.31–.32 (AOU scale) with ARAT r = −.26 to −.33 (QOM scale) with 9-Hole Peg Test r = −.16 to −.023 (AOU scale) with 9-Hole Peg Test r = −.52 (QOM scale) with BBT r = −0.37 to −.49 (AOU scale) with BBT	15–20 minutes
SIS, Hand Function and ADL subscales	Tries to capture real-world abilities from fewer questions; subject to self-report biases	Test–retest = .70–.92	r = 0.57–.73 with ARAT r = 0.61–.83 with Jebsen–Taylor Test of Hand Function r = 0.53–.66 with 9-Hole Peg Test	5 minutes per subscale

Note. One measure from each category can be selected for use. ADL = activities of daily living; AOU =Amount of Use; ARAT = Action Research Arm Test; BBT = Box and Block Test; CAHAI = Chedoke Arm and Hand Activity Inventory; MAL = Motor Activity Log; MI = Motricity Index; NA = not available; QOM = Quality of Movement; SIS = Stroke Impact Scale.

Tyson, 2012). In addition, the ARAT allows observation of various types of grasping and pinching, providing excellent information on which components of movement need to be practiced during task-specific training. Several features of the ARAT and BBT make them feasible to use in clinical practice:

- Administration time is between 5 and 15 minutes, making them quick to perform.
- They are relatively inexpensive and are both commercially available.
- No specialized training is required to perform either assessment.

- Both assessments are portable and can be easily transported to the client for testing.

Self-Report Measures

Motor Activity Log

The Motor Activity Log (MAL; Uswatte, Taub, Morris, Light, & Thompson, 2006; Uswatte, Taub, Morris, Vignolo, & McCulloch, 2005) is a structured interview designed to measure real-world arm use. Clients rate their performance on the basis of how much and how well the affected arm is used to complete a variety of activities in daily life. The measure has two scales, and scores on both range from 0 to 5. The Quality of Movement scale asks clients to rate how well they are able to perform a specific activity, and the Amount of Use scale asks clients to rate how much they use their affected arm to perform the activity. Scores are calculated by averaging the scored items on each scale. Average scores closer to 5 indicate better self-perceived quality of movement or amount of use of the affected arm. The MAL is reliable and valid to use with the stroke population, it takes approximately 15 to 20 minutes to administer, and it can be obtained online.

Stroke Impact Scale

The Stroke Impact Scale (SIS; Duncan, Bode, Min Lai, & Perera, 2003; Duncan, Wallace, Studenski, Lai, & Johnson, 2001; Duncan et al., 1999) is a stroke-specific, self-report measure designed to measure stroke outcomes in the domains of strength, hand function, activities of daily living (ADLs) and instrumental activities of daily living (IADLs), mobility, communication, emotion, memory and thinking, and participation. Questions can be administered face to face, over the phone, or by mail (Duncan, Lai, et al., 2002; Duncan, Reker, et al., 2002). Clients rate their ability on each item on a scale ranging from 1 to 5. Both the Hand Function and the ADL subscales of the SIS are most relevant for measuring UE function. The SIS is reliable and valid to use in the stroke population, takes roughly 5 minutes per domain to administer, and can be obtained online.

In addition to the assessments discussed in detail in this manual, other functional assessments are available for UE evaluation in clinical settings. Other assessments include the Wolf Motor Function Test (Wolf et al., 2001), 9-Hole Peg Test (Mathiowetz, Weber, Kashman, & Volland, 1985), Jebsen–Taylor Test of Hand Function (Jebsen, Taylor, Trieschmann, Trotter, & Howard, 1969), and the Chedoke Arm and Hand Activity Inventory (Barreca et al., 2004, 2006; Barreca, Stratford, Lambert, Masters, & Streiner, 2005). All of these assessments have good reliability and validity and either are available commercially or can be built from published manuals or Web sites. Many of these assessments are highly correlated and could reasonably be chosen for use over the ARAT or the BBT, because they measure the same constructs. A clinician may use whatever functional assessment is available in the clinic, but it is important to use the same assessment both at the initial evaluation and at progress and discharge evaluation to easily determine whether task-specific training is improving outcomes as intended.

Identifying and Setting Goals

Identifying and setting meaningful goals for treatment can often be difficult. One critical issue is that people receiving rehabilitation services may have difficulty participating fully in the goal-setting process (Leach, Cornwell, Fleming, & Haines, 2010). This difficulty may, in part, be due to the type of goal-setting approach used by clinicians (Leach et al., 2010). Contemporary stroke rehabilitation practice guidelines state that interventions should be rooted in functional goals (Duncan et al., 2005; U.S. Department of Defense & U.S. Department of Veterans Affairs, 2010). However, goals often are set at the level of impairment (e.g., "Mr. X will demonstrate left-finger extension range of motion to 20° within 2 weeks") rather than at the level of function (e.g., "Mr. X will independently turn a doorknob to open and close door with left hand within 2 weeks").

It is valuable to use a standardized goal-setting measure such as the Canadian Occupational Performance Measure (COPM; Law et al., 1990; see also Cup, Scholte op Reimer, Thijssen, & van Kuyk-Minis, 2003; Dedding, Cardol, Eyssen, Dekker, & Beelen, 2004; Eyssen et al., 2011) in conjunction with the impairment and function measures described earlier. Use of the COPM, or another similar tool, allows the person receiving services to explicitly state in which activities he or she wants to improve. In addition, for individualized, functional goal setting to occur, the clinician, client, and family need to be involved in the process.

Another critical issue for goal setting is that goals need to be functional activities that the client realistically will be capable of achieving. A substantial amount of data have been published regarding prediction of functional outcomes for people with stroke. These data can be used to determine a client's prognosis. Interestingly, the same pattern of recovery can be seen around the world, whether the data were collected in the United States (Duncan, Lai, & Keighley, 2000) or in Europe (Kwakkel, Kollen, & Lindeman, 2004). In general, these data indicate that the more mild the impairments are at initial presentation (e.g., high Motricity Index score, capable of producing grip and pinch force), the more likely it is that the person will recover dexterity of the upper limb (Beebe & Lang, 2009a; Kwakkel, Kollen, van der Grond, & Prevo, 2003; Nijland, van Wegen, Harmeling-van der Wel, & Kwakkel, 2010). Consistent with this finding, the more severe the symptoms are at initial presentation (e.g., low Motricity Index score, not capable of producing grip or pinch force), the less likely it is that the person will recover motion or dexterity of the upper limb.

Most recovery for people with mild impairments occurs in the first month post stroke, whereas for people with more moderate and severe impairments, the majority of recovery will be complete by 3 months (Jorgensen et al., 1995). In addition, some evidence has emerged for a 10% improvement rule (Lazar et al., 2010; Prabhakaran et al., 2008; Zarahn et al., 2011). This rule suggests that people will improve about 10% on a clinical impairment scale. Obviously, 10% of a bigger number is greater than 10% of a smaller number. Thus, people who are more mildly affected will improve a greater amount than people who are more severely affected.

The implication of these prognostic data for task-specific training is that the clinician needs to make a realistic decision as to the role that the affected UE will play in daily life (e.g., nonfunctional, supportive, dexterous). This decision can then be discussed with the client and family, goals can be set accordingly, and task-specific training can be implemented to achieve the desired goals.

A third critical issue for goal setting is that most daily actions involve both UEs, not just one (Bailey & Lang, in press). Bilateral tasks may require symmetrical use of the extremities, in which both extremities are doing the same amount of work and making the same movements (e.g., lifting a pan onto a shelf), or asymmetrical use of the extremities, in which the extremities are working to execute a task but have different roles (e.g., opening a jug of milk with one hand holding the jug and the other hand unscrewing the lid). It is therefore appropriate to select goals, and subsequent activities to practice, that require the use of both extremities.

For a client with moderate to severe paresis, it may be best to select tasks for which the affected hand is the supporting hand, acting as the stabilizer providing gross assistance, while the unaffected hand is the "doer," or the hand that actively completes the dexterous portion of the task. For example, when carrying a stack of towels, a person can place the affected hand on top of the stack to stabilize it and the unaffected hand underneath the stack to support its weight. In addition, if little return of distal strength and fine motor control is expected, goals may be centered around proximal limb control instead of distal (e.g., using the limb to assist with wiping down tables). The goals of task-specific training may be focused on training the affected UE to be the supportive hand or training it to be the dexterous hand. Chapter 3, "Task-Specific Training," provides examples of matching assessment results to goals and tasks practiced.

Summary

UE assessment is important for determining the initial level of impairment, function, and activity. Comparing assessment results with the client's rehabilitation goals helps determine whether goals are achievable or need adjustment. Assessment results then guide interventions to achieve the client's goals.

CHAPTER 3

Task-Specific Training

Matching Goals With Specific Tasks

After collecting the assessment information and goals, the next step is to match the goals to specific tasks. Table 3.1 provides examples of goals that could be generated from the Canadian Occupational Performance Measure (COPM; Law et al., 1990), some tasks that could be practiced during therapy sessions, and the rationale for their selection.

Clients may identify many different goals as they participate in rehabilitation. No single "correct" task addresses each goal. Figures 3.1–3.3 provide examples of three individual cases of matching COPM goals to assessment results and to a chosen task and how to grade that task. This situation is one in which the practitioner can use his or her creative side to coordinate what the client practices in therapy with what the client wants to be able to do outside of therapy. When setting goals,

- Encourage clients to select goals that are measurable and related to a functional task. For example, "return to gardening, using both hands" is a more appropriate choice than "make my right arm better." Clients may need to be redirected during goal setting to ensure that the goals match the therapy services being provided.
- Encourage goals that match the expected prognosis. If the client is within the first few weeks post stroke and has movement in all joints (Motricity Index [MI; Collin & Wade, 1990] scores >50), set goals anticipating the return of dexterous ability to the affected upper extremity (UE). If the client is approximately 3 months or more post stroke, set goals that anticipate small improvements. If, once beyond the first 3 to 4 weeks post stroke, the client has minimal movement (MI scores <50), set goals anticipating that the affected hand will be the supportive hand.

When matching goals to tasks,

- Make every attempt to have clients perform the whole task during the training (see principles in Table 1.1). In cases in which whole-task practice is not realistic (e.g., too complicated, insufficient equipment or environment, insufficient motor abilities), part of the task could be chosen instead. When splitting a task into parts, keep the parts as natural as possible and do not make artificial breaks in the activity. Remind the client that the part he or she is practicing is going to lead to the ability to perform the whole task, and encourage progression to whole-task performance as soon as possible.
- Include tasks that have multiple movement components (see Chapter 1, "Overview of Task-Specific Training"), because everyday UE function requires such components strung together in different ways. In the example of scrapbooking (see Table 3.1, last row), the actions of cutting, gluing, and manipulating different-sized photographs all require reaching, grasping, moving or manipulating, and then releasing objects. It is critical to practice all of the movement components and preferable to practice them in a functional sequence.

Grading Tasks to Challenge Motor Capabilities

Information on motor capabilities comes from the impairment and function assessments (see Chapter 2, "Assessment for Task-Specific Training"), so selected tasks should be graded to match the client's motor capabilities. Do not simply repeat tasks that the person is already skilled at accomplishing, and do not select tasks that he or she has repeatedly failed to perform. Tasks should challenge but not overwhelm or under-

Table 3.1. Examples of Goals, Tasks Chosen to Address Them, and Rationales for Their Choice

Goal	Tasks Chosen to Address the Goal	Rationale for Chosen Task
Improve handwriting	Practice writing; incrementally write faster or write to improve quality and accuracy.	Handwriting is necessary to sign documents and to complete work duties. Manipulating a pen addresses distal strength and fine motor control.
Improve typing speed and accuracy	Practice typing; incrementally type faster or type longer words.	Typing is often necessary for work, including communication (e.g., e-mail), and addresses distal strength and motor control.
Return to fishing	Pick up fishing lures; sort a tackle box; cast a fishing line.	Fishing is an important leisure activity for many people. Manipulating fishing-related equipment addresses fine motor control, and larger movements such as casting address proximal and distal motor control and strength.
Be able to play games with grandchildren	Play Connect Four™; deal cards.	Playing social games is an important leisure activity for many people. Different games of interest to the client can be selected to address motor impairments of the proximal or distal UE.
Be able to fold towels as part of laundry chores	Fold towels or washcloths.	Folding is a bilateral activity and an integral part of many household tasks. Grasping and releasing clothing is also important for dressing.
Safely place and remove objects onto shelves	Lift cans to or remove cans from shelves.	This task mimics many common daily movements such as unloading a grocery bag and retrieving craft or hobby supplies. It can be graded to address proximal and distal motor impairments.
Safely empty silverware from dishwasher	Pick up silverware and sort into container.	Silverware is used at most meals. This activity addresses grasp and release of objects.
Readily hold and manipulate coins	Pick up a variety of coins and place in a piggy bank with a coin slot.	Manipulation of money is an everyday task and addresses fine motor control.
Return to scrapbooking	Cut paper with scissors.	Scrapbooking is a common leisure activity, involving cutting, pasting or gluing, and manipulating different-sized papers and photographs. The variety of movements required can be structured to address proximal and distal motor impairments.

Note. UE = upper extremity.

whelm each client's motor capabilities, referred to as the "just-right" challenge (Rebeiro & Polgar, 1999). To optimize progress, a client must be able to recognize what needs to be accomplished (what the task is) and feel capable of achieving that task. Once the task is achieved (i.e., learned), the task difficulty is increased to continue improving performance (Rebeiro & Polgar, 1999). Using the goals of the COPM and the following rules helps to achieve the just-right challenge:

- It is okay if the client does not perform the task perfectly and has many failures.

- The task must be sufficiently challenging to require the client to problem solve ways to complete it.
- As a guideline, a single repetition of a task at the just-right challenge should take approximately 6 to 15 seconds. These numbers are based on observations of people practicing UE task-specific training in our laboratory (Birkenmeier, Prager, & Lang, 2010).
- Performance of the task does not have to look good. Depending on the time since the stroke and the severity of paresis, allowing and prac-

Figure 3.1. Matching goals to assessment results and task selection and grading: Client with limited upper-extremity function.

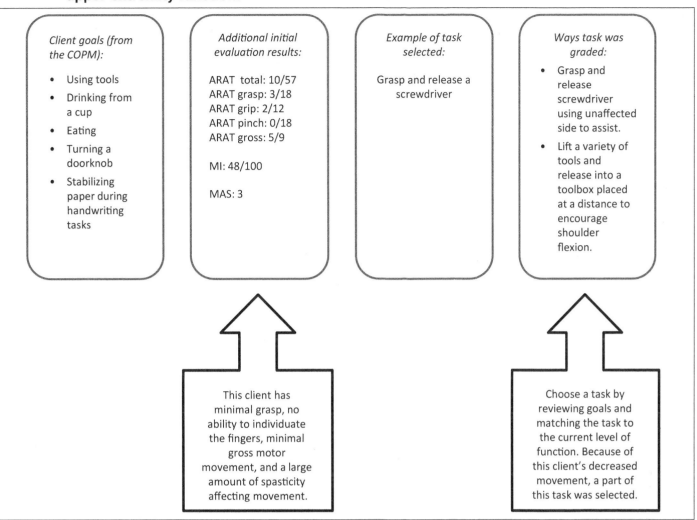

Note. ARAT = Action Research Arm Test; COPM = Canadian Occupational Performance Measure; MAS = Molar Assessment Scale; MI = Motricity Index.

ticing compensatory movements to accomplish functional tasks is often appropriate. If the goal of rehabilitation is to improve UE function, then it may be a disservice to focus on unrealistic, ideal movement patterns. In the case of mildly paretic clients early after stroke when compensatory movements are not desired, the practitioner is encouraged to set up the training experience to promote the desired movement patterns and strategies rather than spending effort providing feedback on quality of movement. For example, if the desired reach pattern is pure shoulder flexion with no abduction during the task of putting cans on shelves, then the practitioner can posi-

tion the client with the reaching arm next to the wall, such that he or she is forced into shoulder flexion to elevate the arm.

After tasks have been chosen, the client attempts to perform each activity. Tasks should be graded to address the underlying movement impairments specific to each client. The practitioner has identified the underlying movement impairments on the basis of individual item scores from the evaluation and observation of movement. For example, if the client could not grasp the large items on the Action Research Arm Test (ARAT; Lyle, 1981), then picking containers that challenge finger extension during grasping is appropriate.

Figure 3.2. Matching goals to assessment results and task selection and grading: Client with moderate upper-extremity function.

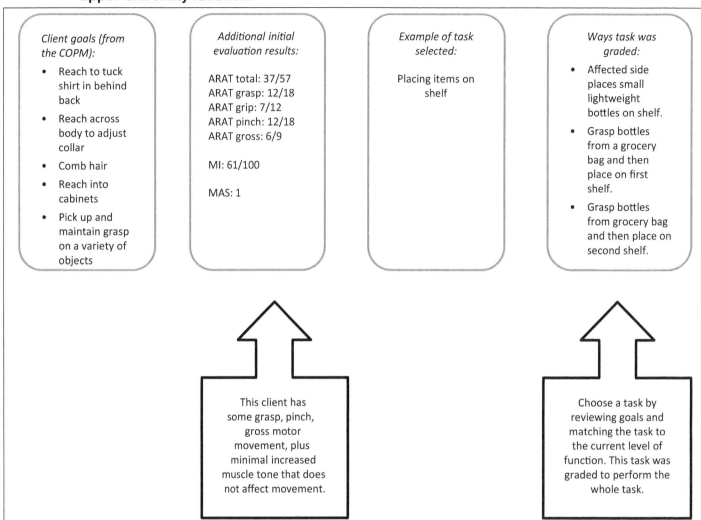

Client goals (from the COPM):	*Additional initial evaluation results:*	*Example of task selected:*	*Ways task was graded:*
• Reach to tuck shirt in behind back • Reach across body to adjust collar • Comb hair • Reach into cabinets • Pick up and maintain grasp on a variety of objects	ARAT total: 37/57 ARAT grasp: 12/18 ARAT grip: 7/12 ARAT pinch: 12/18 ARAT gross: 6/9 MI: 61/100 MAS: 1	Placing items on shelf	• Affected side places small lightweight bottles on shelf. • Grasp bottles from a grocery bag and then place on first shelf. • Grasp bottles from grocery bag and then place on second shelf.

This client has some grasp, pinch, gross motor movement, plus minimal increased muscle tone that does not affect movement.

Choose a task by reviewing goals and matching the task to the current level of function. This task was graded to perform the whole task.

Note. ARAT = Action Research Arm Test; COPM = Canadian Occupational Performance Measure; MAS = Molar Assessment Scale; MI = Motricity Index.

The practitioner's skill is in ensuring that the goals and assessment scores are matched to training tasks.

Next, we provide an example of how goals, assessment results, tasks, and grading are all linked together. A woman with decreased proximal strength (a score of <3 of 5 on manual muscle testing, <60 on the UE MI, or both) and decreased fine motor control (good finger opposition but difficulty maintaining a tip-to-tip pinch grip; ARAT pinch = 12 of 18) who also enjoys playing games with her grandchildren (per her COPM goals) might practice the task of playing Connect Four. During the first attempts at this task, the client can be seated with the game grid placed directly in front of her, on nonslip material to prevent slipping.

Success would be indicated by the client's consistently picking up the colored disc on the first attempt and releasing it accurately into a slot. The practitioner would be able to tell whether this task was sufficiently challenging by whether the client frequently requires multiple attempts to pick up the disc, the client frequently drops the disc before reaching the grid, or the disc is not dropped into the grid. As the client improves, she should require less time to complete the same number of repetitions (e.g., drops 80 discs in the grid in 8 minutes instead of 14 minutes). Also as the client improves, the grid can be moved further away from her body, challenging her to produce more shoulder elevation and elbow extension.

Figure 3.3. Matching goals to assessment results and task selection and grading: Client with higher upper-extremity function.

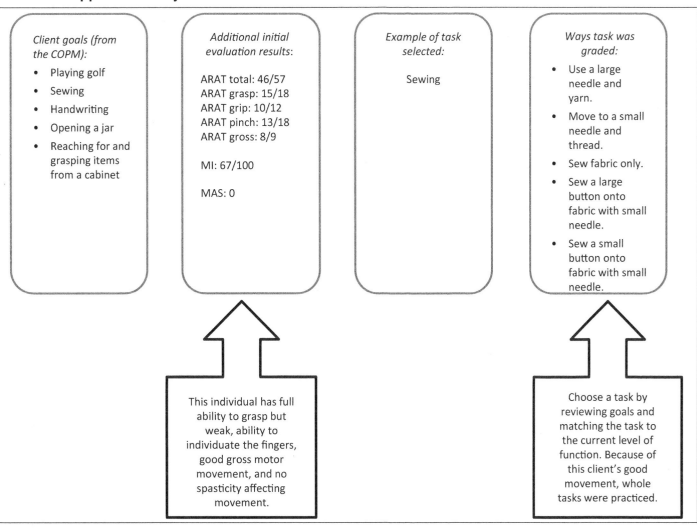

Note. ARAT = Action Research Arm Test; COPM = Canadian Occupational Performance Measure; MAS = Molar Assessment Scale; MI = Motricity Index.

This area is another in which the creative practitioner will excel in implementing task-specific training, because the task can be set up in many ways to make it challenging for the client. Table 3.2 provides a list of universal ways to make tasks harder (grade up) or easier (grade down). Note that it often takes experimentation with the client and the task to find the just-right challenge.

Progressing or Changing Tasks

Grading Up

What does the practitioner do when the client's performance on a task reaches a plateau or the task seems too easy? It is time to progress the task and make it harder. In other words, the task needs to be graded up. Several different criteria can be used in deciding when to grade a task up. Exhibit 3.1 provides several suggestions for when it might be the right time to make the task harder. If the answer to one or more of the questions is yes, then it is likely time to make the task harder.

Other "what-if" situations when grading up include

- *What if the grade-up does not result in very much change?* Continue to make the task harder until the client is successfully being challenged, for example, the answers to the questions in Exhibit 3.1 are all no.

Table 3.2. Universal Grading Techniques

Way to Change the Grade of the Task	General Direction of Difficulty
Changing the physical position of the client	Standing = harder Sitting = easier
Changing the position of task materials: height, depth, location	Higher,[a] deeper on the table, and further away from midline = harder Lower,[a] closer on the table, and closer to midline = easier
Changing the weight of task materials	Heavy objects = harder Light objects = easier
Changing the size of objects	Larger items = harder Smaller items = easier
Using adaptive equipment and materials	Stabilize objects with nonslip material = easier Increase grip surface of object (e.g., built-up pen) = easier Other adaptive equipment = easier

[a]Reverse the difficulty if reaching from waist level downward.

- *What if the client is ready to be graded up on all the tasks he or she practices in a session?* Make the most critical tasks harder, but keep at least one the same. If every task is graded up at the same time, the client could easily become overwhelmed and overtired. Plan ahead to grade up different tasks at different times.
- *What if the client has been training on the task for many sessions and is not getting better at it?* If performance is not changing at all (i.e., the client is still dropping the item as frequently, not getting any faster, still having trouble reaching to the same height, taking the same amount of time to complete the same number of repetitions), then it may be time to switch tasks. The unchanging performance suggests that the client is not mastering this task. The clinician can decide to switch to a different task that trains similar movements or to abandon the goal of completing this task and focus on other tasks.
- *Should the client stick with the same tasks throughout the duration of therapy services?* The general goal of most UE task-specific training programs is to improve UE function in everyday life. It is impossible, however, to practice all UE tasks that a person needs to perform within the typical time allotted for therapy services. To increase the likelihood that training will transfer to other tasks, it is important to switch tasks periodically. Tasks can be switched to address other goals (e.g., fishing vs. handwriting; see Table 3.1) or can be switched to address other

Exhibit 3.1. Questions to Determine Whether It Is Time to Grade Up (i.e., Make a Task Harder)

Question	Yes	No
• Can the client complete the task successfully 90% of the time (e.g., not dropping object, grasping object on first attempt, placing and releasing object in correct location on the first attempt)?	☐	☐
• Has the client stated that the task is too easy and that he or she is not being challenged? (Feel free to ask the client this question.)	☐	☐
• Does the client take only a short time to complete the assigned or desired repetitions (e.g., a single repetition takes <3 seconds or it takes ≤10 minutes for 100 repetitions)?	☐	☐
• Does the client report being satisfied with how he or she is performing the task?	☐	☐

actions that need to be completed to accomplish the goal (e.g., within the goal of returning to fishing, reeling vs. organizing tackle box).

Grading Down

What does the practitioner do when the task is too difficult for the client? In most instances, tasks are made easier, or graded down, less frequently than they are made harder, or graded up. Two scenarios occur in which it is most common to grade a task down: (1) The task has been graded up too much and is too difficult or (2) the client is having an off day (e.g., unusually emotional, overly fatigued), and the task needs to be made easier for a brief time. As with grading up, criteria exist that can be used in deciding when to grade a task down. Exhibit 3.2 contains several suggestions for when it might be the right time to grade down the task. If the client answers yes to one or more of the questions in Exhibit 3.2, then it is likely appropriate to make the task easier.

Other "what-if" situations when grading down include

- *What if the client wants to work or continue working on a task the clinician feels is too hard?* Working on goals that are meaningful to the client is a priority of task-specific training. Consider negotiating with the client to practice a slightly easier version of the task with the promise of moving up to the more difficult version soon.
- *What if the client reports the task is too hard or gets frustrated during the task?* Grade the task down if the client is performing 50% or fewer of the desired repetitions, or consider switching tasks if the task is no longer motivating to the client.
- *What if the client reports extreme fatigue or has other medical considerations affecting performance during a treatment session?* Temporarily grade the task down to a level appropriate for the client's performance for the day. Return to the pre-event level (not the graded-down level) at the next treatment session. Conditions to consider include low blood sugar associated with diabetes, fluctuating spasticity, decreased sleep or lack of sleep, other life stressors, and so forth. Continue to monitor the client's medical status throughout the treatment session (e.g., respiratory rate, heart rate, blood pressure, subjective feelings).

How to grade a task up or down can be determined on the basis of the underlying movement impairments. For example, a client who is ready to grade up on the task of lifting cans to a shelf and has difficulty extending the fingers will be progressed to a wider can to challenge finger extension. Likewise, another client who is ready to grade up on the same task but has difficulty producing sufficient grip force will be progressed to a heavier can to challenge grip force production.

Changing to New or Different Tasks

Changing to new or different tasks is inevitable. It is highly likely that a client will tire of doing the same tasks for weeks in a row, thus making it practical to switch to other tasks. These guidelines may help the

---

Exhibit 3.2. Questions to Determine Whether It Is Time to Grade Down (i.e., Make a Task Easier)

Question	Yes	No
• Is the client completing ≤50% of the assigned or desired repetitions for a given task?	☐	☐
• Does the client exhibit extreme frustration during the task?	☐	☐
• Does the client take a long time to achieve the assigned or desired repetitions (e.g., a single repetition takes >30 seconds, it takes ≥20 minutes for 100 repetitions)?	☐	☐
• Does the client exhibit extreme fatigue during the task or is the client unable perform the task at all? (*Extreme fatigue* or *inability to perform* is operationally defined as 10 consecutive failures to complete a particular task.)	☐	☐

practitioner decide when it is the right time to make a task switch:

- *The task is no longer challenging to the client.* Suggestions for change: Select a new task using previously identified goals when the client is able to perform the whole activity without difficulty.
- *The client wants to practice reaching, grasping, moving, or manipulating in the context of a different task.* Suggestions for change: At the beginning of a new treatment week, pick one new task related to previously identified goals.
- *The client states that he or she does not like a treatment activity.* Suggestions for change: Evaluate the current treatment task to determine which movements were being addressed with the disliked task, and select another task to work on the same movements. Again, use previously identified goals.

A necessary and important part of rehabilitation is documentation of therapy services. In many settings, clients are seen by multiple practitioners over the course of treatment. As with any intervention, it is critical that the delivery of task-specific training be easily implemented by all staff. Systematic documentation of each treatment session will assist with this. It is important to record the task, the way the task is set up, and the way the task is graded. Exhibits 3.3 and 3.4 provide sample daily documentation forms to track what is occurring during therapy sessions and how. After each blank form is an example of a completed form. Although these forms will not work for every situation, they provide a starting point for practitioners or facilities to create their own paper or electronic forms to track task-specific training.

Feedback During Training

Learning requires solving the motor problem, not rote repetition of overlearned tasks (see Table 1.1). Thus, it is important to allow the client to problem solve throughout the task to determine the strategies that are most beneficial for task completion. In animal experiments of motor learning and plasticity, no one tells the animal how to move correctly or how to complete the task; the animal figures it out by itself. This same idea applies to task-specific training.

Clinicians often feel as though the value added is in the specific feedback about how to move. Experimental learning results suggest the opposite is true, however. Explicit feedback can often slow the rate of motor learning (Boyd & Winstein, 2006). Too much information can distract the learner from important internal feedback. Because the practitioner spends time with the client only during therapy sessions, it is logical that the client will develop his or her own sense of what movements or strategies will and will not work for movement in everyday life.

In task-specific training, clinicians' skill shines when the goals are matched to the training task, the tasks are creatively implemented to produce functional gains, and the client is allowed to seek out his or her own successful movement strategies.

Summary

Matching goals with specific tasks, grading tasks to challenge motor capabilities, and progressing and changing tasks as needed are crucial aspects of task-specific training.

Exhibit 3.3. Daily Documentation Form: Task-Specific Training Summary Page and Example

Client: _____   Date: _____

Practitioner: _____

REPETITIONS

Total Repetitions Task 1: _____

Total Repetitions Task 2: _____

Total Repetitions Task 3: _____

Total Repetitions Completed for Session: _____

MINUTES ON TASK

Total Minutes Task 1: _____

Total Minutes Task 2: _____

Total Minutes Task 3: _____

Total Minutes Completed for Session: _____

Comments:

(Continued)

Exhibit 3.3. Daily Documentation Form: Task-Specific Training Summary Page and Example *(Cont.)*

Name: John Smith   **Date:** 1/1/2014

Practitioner Name: R. Birkenmeier, OTD, OTR/L

REPETITIONS

Total Repetitions Task 1: 98

Total Repetitions Task 2: 103

Total Repetitions Task 3: 100

Total Repetitions Completed for Session: 301

MINUTES ON TASK

Total Minutes Task 1: 17:49

Total Minutes Task 2: 18:25

Total Minutes Task 3: 18:37

Total Minutes Completed for Session: 54:11

Comments:

Mr. Smith c/o shoulder pain at the beginning of the session. He rated his pain as 6/10.
Mr. Smith stated his shoulder pain decreased at the end of the session. He rated his pain as 2/10.

Exhibit 3.4. Task-Specific Training Documentation Page and Example

Client: _____ Date: _____

Practitioner: _____

Repetitions	Minutes of Training
Total Repetitions Task # _____:	Total Minutes Task # _____:
_____	_____

Task: _____

Task Description and Grading:

_____

_____

_____

_____

1	2	3	4	5	6	7	8	9	10	11	12	13	14	15	16	17	18	19	20

21	22	23	24	25	26	27	28	29	30	31	32	33	34	35	36	37	38	39	40

41	42	43	44	45	46	47	48	49	50	51	52	53	54	55	56	57	58	59	60

61	62	63	64	65	66	67	68	69	70	71	72	73	74	75	76	77	78	79	80

81	82	83	84	85	86	87	88	89	90	91	92	93	94	95	96	97	98	99	100

(Continued)

Exhibit 3.4. Task-Specific Training Documentation Page and Example *(Cont.)*

Name: John Smith   **Date:** 1/1/2014

Practitioner Name: R. Birkenmeier, OTD, OTR/L

Repetitions	Minutes of Training
Total Repetitions Task 1:	Total Minutes Task 1:
98	17:49

Task Name: Pouring juice into a cup

Task Description and Grading:

Seated at table with orange juice jug filled with water and 2 plastic cups on table. Grab jug with affected RUE and pour a small amount into 1 cup, then release grip and set jug down. Then grasp and pour a small amount of water into another cup. After cups are full, empty cups, refill juice jug with water, and continue until desired amount of repetitions is achieved.

1 grasp, pour, release of jug = 1 rep

1	2	3	4	5	6	7	8	9	10	11	12	13	14	15	16	17	18	19	20

21	22	23	24	25	26	27	28	29	30	31	32	33	34	35	36	37	38	39	40

41	42	43	44	45	46	47	48	49	50	51	52	53	54	55	56	57	58	59	60

61	62	63	64	65	66	67	68	69	70	71	72	73	74	75	76	77	78	79	80

81	82	83	84	85	86	87	88	89	90	91	92	93	94	95	96	97	98	99	100

Toolbox of Upper-Extremity Tasks

It is important that clinicians select tasks that are meaningful to the clients performing them. Higher levels of motivation and engagement may be obtained when task selection is aligned with client goals (see Table 1.1 in Chapter 1, "Principles to Guide Task-Specific Training").

This chapter consists of 100 tasks, with descriptions of how the task may be executed and modified for clients with varying levels of impairment. The purpose of this chapter is to give clinicians a quick reference to aid in selecting an appropriate task for any client. Each task consists of the following parts:

- Key impairments addressed,
- Materials needed,
- Task description,
- Ideas to upgrade or downgrade the task,
- Ways to determine whether the task is mastered, and
- Ideas for related taskss.

Tasks

The tasks are organized into the following categories: self-care, productivity, and leisure (Exhibit 4.1, "Categorical Index of Tasks"). An alphabetical index (Exhibit 4.2, "Alphabetical Index of Tasks") is also provided. Both indices list each task with the verb first, followed by the noun. The following scenarios demonstrate how to navigate the categorical and alphabetical indices:

- *Scenario 1:* A client would like to return to playing card games with his friends. The clinician would turn to the Leisure section of the categorical index and find the task "playing cards." This task can also be found in the alphabetical index.
- *Scenario 2:* A client has difficulty verbalizing his goals, but his wife states that it takes him a long time to tie his shoes. The client agrees that he

would like to work on this issue. The clinician would find "tying shoes" under Self-care in the categorical index or in the alphabetical index.
- *Scenario 3:* A client states that she makes many errors when typing e-mails on her computer at work. The clinician suggests that typing be included in her treatment plan. The clinician would search in the Productivity section of the categorical index for "typing" or find it in the alphabetical index.
- *Scenario 4:* A client would like to work on getting dressed. The clinician would find specific tasks such as "tying shoes," "zipping jacket," "donning and doffing socks," and so forth in the categorical index under Self-care or in the alphabetical index.
- *Scenario 5:* A client would like to practice doing laundry. The clinician would search for related tasks in the Productivity section of the categorical index or in the alphabetical index: such as "folding towels," "hanging clothes on hangers," "stacking laundry," "pouring detergent into washing machine," and so forth.
- *Scenario 6:* A client would like to practice eating. The clinician would search in the Self-care section in the categorical index or in the alphabetical index for tasks such as "cutting food," "eating soup," "drinking from a cup," and so forth.

Key Impairments Addressed

Each task includes a list of the key upper-extremity (UE) movement impairments that it addresses (see Exhibits 4.3–4.5). The terms chosen to describe the impairments are general and are consistent with patterns of weakness observed in people poststroke (Beebe & Lang, 2008; Bohannon & Smith, 1987b; Lang & Beebe, 2007). These terms include *decreased proximal strength, decreased distal strength, decreased*

Exhibit 4.1. Categorical Index of Tasks

Self-care

Clipping fingernails 32
Washing body 33
Tying shoes 34
Brushing hair 35
Zipping jacket 36
Folding socks 37
Brushing teeth 38
Eating soup 39
Donning and doffing jacket 40
Drinking from cup 41
Applying bandage 42
Unwrapping piece of candy 43
Grasping shoes from shoebox 44
Filing fingernails 45
Donning and doffing socks 46
Opening and closing umbrella 47
Pumping soap from dispenser 48
Washing hair 49
Donning and doffing eyeglasses 50
Donning wristwatch 51
Shaving face 52
Applying deodorant 53
Donning and doffing gloves 54

Productivity

Typing 55
Handwriting 56
Clicking computer mouse 57
Counting money 58
Organizing toolbox 59
Navigating digital tablet or
    e-reader 60
Sewing 61
Flipping light switch 62
Cutting food 63
Removing lids 64
Removing towels from laundry
    basket 65

Folding towels 66
Hanging clothes on hangers 67
Placing cans on shelf 68
Sweeping floor 69
Opening door 70
Drying pots and pans 71
Sanding wall 72
Sorting silverware 73
Answering telephone 74
Assembling nut and bolt 75
Driving screw into wood 76
Fastening paperclip to papers 77
Filling out forms 78
Locking door 79
Placing coins into vending
    machine 80
Retrieving wallet from pocket 81
Retrieving bills from billfold 82
Dialing telephone number 83
Turning steering wheel 84
Turning oven dial or timer 85
Fastening clothes to clothesline 86
Opening containers 87
Pouring cereal from box 88
Opening resealable plastic bag 89
Tying grocery bag 90
Packing and unpacking backpack 91
Tacking paper to bulletin board 92
Dusting table 93
Stacking laundry 94
Stacking books on bookshelf 95
Chopping vegetables 96
Emptying trash can 97
Placing trash bag into trash can 98
Grasping paper towel from roll 99
Donning headphones 100
Spreading peanut butter
    onto bread 101
Using calculator 102

Wrapping food in foil 103
Setting microwave 104
Squeezing dish soap from bottle 105
Pouring detergent into
    dishwasher 106
Pouring detergent into
    washing machine 107
Adjusting rearview mirror in car 108
Slicing pizza 109
Peeling vegetables 110
Placing cookie sheet into oven 111
Mailing a letter 112
Fastening twist tie to bread bag 113
Using rolling pin 114
Raking leaves 115
Watering plants 116

Leisure

Casting fishing line 117
Scrapbooking 118
Rolling dice 119
Playing cards 120
Bowling 121
Placing DVD into DVD player 122
Turning pages of book 123
Playing Connect Four 124
Threading beads onto necklace 125
Playing bingo 126
Swinging tennis racquet 127
Planting flowers 128
Golfing 129
Lighting candle 130
Taking photo 131

Exhibit 4.2. Alphabetical Index of Tasks

grip strength, decreased pinch grip, decreased proximal motor control, decreased distal motor control, and *decreased fine motor control.* Following are explanations of the seven terms (in bold), including more specific terms that fall into each category. (*Note.* Impairments in active range of motion are not listed because they are synonymous with the strength impairments [i.e., both common clinical terms reflect paresis].)

1. **Decreased proximal strength,** which includes
   - Decreased scapular or scapulohumeral strength
   - Decreased shoulder flexion or extension strength
   - Decreased shoulder abduction or adduction strength
   - Decreased shoulder internal or external rotation
   - Decreased elbow flexion or extension strength.
   For example, it is common for strength deficits to be similar in muscles of the arm and shoulder as well as the scapula. *Decreased proximal strength* describes weakness at these structures in all planes of movement.
2. **Decreased distal strength,** which includes
   - Decreased forearm pronation or supination strength
   - Decreased wrist flexion or extension strength
   - Decreased radial or ulnar deviation strength
   - Decreased gross finger flexion or extension strength.
   For example, it is common for a person who has decreased strength in his or her wrist flexors and extensors to also have decreased strength in his or her finger flexors and extensors. Therefore, the general impairment decreased distal strength encompasses forearm, wrist, and finger weakness.
3. **Decreased grip strength,** defined as decreased finger flexion strength for gripping
4. **Decreased pinch grip,** defined as decreased index finger and thumb opposition strength
5. **Decreased proximal motor control,** defined as decreased coordination of the UE resulting from lack of motor control at the shoulder, elbow, or both
6. **Decreased distal motor control,** defined as decreased coordination of the UE resulting from

lack of motor control at the forearm, wrist, or hand
7. **Decreased fine motor control,** defined as decreased coordination of the fingers.

The clinician's initial assessment of the UE will help him or her determine the client's initial level of impairment. The clinician may then refer to the key impairment list included with each task example to find the most appropriate task that not only is consistent with the client's goal but also addresses the client's specific UE impairments. The impairment lists are not exhaustive; however, they highlight the primary sensorimotor impairments that make the movements required to execute the tasks challenging.

Materials

Materials needed to complete the task are listed. The client's safety and well-being must be a top priority when selecting materials to carry out tasks. For example, the clinician should consider using candy as a substitute for pills when the client is practicing medication management. If a client is practicing shaving, the clinician should keep the cap on the razor. If a client has a goal of placing dishes in a cupboard, the clinician should consider using plastic or paper dishes instead of breakable dishes.

It is best to be prepared with all the necessary materials before a treatment session. The clinician can anticipate the need for adaptive materials and have easy access to supplies such as cylindrical foam, nonslip material, and tape so a task can be quickly modified to increase or decrease the challenge for the client. An additional hint to make the training session flow smoothly is to have multiple objects in readily countable increments. If the clinician has 10 containers ready, then it is easy to count repetitions by 10s when all the containers have been opened.

Task Description

Within each example is a description of how to execute the task. The clinician must use good judgment with regard to supervising the client to prevent falls while a task is being performed. The clinician must provide the necessary level of assistance to or guarding for the client with compromised balance during a standing or dynamic sitting activity. The task descriptions are written under the assumption that the client will be performing 100 or more repetitions of the task within a certain time constraint.

Grading Task

Tasks are graded to match the client's motor capabilities (see Chapter 3, "Task-Specific Training"). For each task, we provide a few examples of how it could be upgraded or downgraded. Please refer to Chapter 3 for guidelines on deciding when to grade a task up or down.

Task Mastery

The next section of each example is Task Mastery, which explains ways in which the clinician may determine whether the client has mastered the task. These ways include, but are not limited to, consistent completion of each repetition without errors (i.e., dropping items), grasping an item correctly on the first attempt, and hitting the target consistently.

Ideas for Related Tasks

The final section of each example includes Ideas for related taskss with a rationale provided for how these tasks are related. The related tasks require similar movement patterns and thus address similar key impairments. For example, a related task under "Retrieving Wallet From Pocket" is "Tucking Shirt in Back of Pants." These tasks are not functionally related, but they both require sufficient shoulder extension and finger flexion and extension to reach behind the back at waist level to complete the task.

Some of the Ideas for related taskss are other example tasks in this manual and some are not. In the instances in which they are not, the clinician is encouraged to apply what has been learned from the manual and create a new task. A blank template is provided in Exhibit 4.6 ("Blank Task Description Form") at the end of the example tasks for this purpose.

Summary

This toolbox of UE tasks contains 100 self-care, productivity, and leisure tasks. Selecting tasks that are meaningful for the client and well-aligned with his or her goals will lead to higher levels of motivation and engagement while addressing key impairments.

Exhibit 4.3. Self-Care Tasks

1. Task: Clipping fingernails

Key Impairments Addressed:
1. Decreased pinch grip
2. Decreased fine motor control

Materials:
Fingernail clippers
Scrap paper or sponge to clip

Task Description:
1. Sit with fingernail clippers on table.
2. Grasp clippers with affected upper extremity and clip paper or sponge.
3. Set clippers down and release grip.

Grading Task:

Increase difficulty	Decrease difficulty
Use smaller clippers. • Requires more fine motor control.	Use larger clippers (i.e., toenail clippers). • Requires less fine motor control.
Clip into firm material. • Requires more pinch grip.	Build up clipper levers • Requires less fine motor control.
	Clip into soft material. • Requires less pinch grip.
Simulate clipping toenails by assuming proper position to reach toenails (i.e., sitting with hip flexed and abducted and ankle resting on opposite knee) and holding paper or sponge at this location. • Requires more attention to body position and upper-extremity posture.	Hold clippers on table or in lap in front of client. • Requires less attention to body position.

Task Mastery:
1. Consistently grasps and releases clippers on first attempt, without dropping.
2. Consistently clips through paper or sponge.
3. Consistently uses proper pinch grip.

Ideas for related tasks	Rationale
Fastening clothespin	Requires pinch grip and fine motor control.
Fastening papers with binder clip	Requires pinch grip and fine motor control.
Closing bag with bag clip	Requires pinch grip and fine motor control.

2. Task: Washing body

Key Impairments Addressed:
1. Decreased proximal strength
2. Decreased grip strength

Materials:
Washcloth or bath mitt

Task Description:
1. Stand with washcloth on table.
2. Grasp washcloth with affected hand and wash opposite arm from hand to shoulder and back down.
3. Replace washcloth on table and release grip.

Grading Task:

Increase difficulty	Decrease difficulty
Stand with washcloth on shelf. • Requires more proximal strength.	Sit with cloth on lap versus table. • Requires less proximal strength.
Use a hand towel. • Requires more grip strength to grasp and hold towel.	Keep a bath mitt on the hand throughout task. • Requires no grip strength.
Wash behind the head or back. • Requires more proximal strength.	Wash the thigh or abdomen. • Requires less proximal strength.

Task Mastery:
1. Consistently grasps washcloth without dropping.
2. Consistently reaches target landmark (i.e., biceps or acromion).

Ideas for related tasks	Rationale
Applying lotion	Requires proximal and distal strength.
Applying deodorant	Requires proximal strength and grip strength.
Drying self off with towel	Requires proximal strength and grip strength.

3. Task: Tying shoes

Key Impairments Addressed:
1. Decreased distal strength
2. Decreased fine motor control

Materials:
Tennis shoe with laces

Task Description:
1. Grasp laces with bilateral hands, cross laces, and tie into bow.
2. Untie with unaffected or affected hand.

Grading Task:

Increase difficulty	Decrease difficulty
Tie shoes with small laces; tie yarn or thread. • Requires more fine motor control	Tie shoes with thick laces; tie a rope. • Requires less fine motor control.
Tie and double knot laces. • Requires more fine motor control.	Only cross laces and pull, no bow. • Requires less fine motor control.
Tie shoes while on feet. • Requires attention to body position and upper-extremity posture.	Tie shoes stabilized in lap or on table. • Requires less attention to body position and upper-extremity posture.

Task Mastery:
1. Does not drop laces.
2. Consistently ties and unties laces on first attempt.

Ideas for related tasks	Rationale
Tying a necktie	Requires distal strength. Requires fine motor control.
Tying drawstring pants	Requires distal strength. Requires fine motor control.

4. Task: Brushing hair

Key Impairments Addressed:
1. Decreased proximal strength
2. Decreased grip strength
3. Decreased proximal motor control

Materials:
Hairbrush or comb

Task Description:
1. Sit with hairbrush on table.
2. Grasp and simulate brushing hair three to four times.
3. Set brush back onto table.

Grading Task:

Increase difficulty	Decrease difficulty
Use hairbrush with a smaller handle. • Requires more distal strength.	Use hairbrush with a larger handle. • Requires less distal strength.
Note. May decrease difficulty depending on client's finger range of motion limitations.	*Note.* May increase difficulty depending on client's finger range of motion limitations.
Simulate brushing the back of the head. • Requires more proximal strength.	Simulate brushing the front or side of the head. • Requires less proximal strength.
Use a heavy hairbrush. • Requires more proximal strength and grip strength.	Use a lightweight hairbrush. • Requires less proximal strength and grip strength.

Task Mastery:
1. Consistently grasps and releases hairbrush without dropping.
2. Consistently reaches target.

Ideas for related tasks	Rationale
Drying hair	Requires proximal strength and grip strength. Requires proximal motor control.
Washing hair	Requires proximal strength and distal strength. Requires proximal motor control.
Styling hair	Requires proximal strength and grip strength. Requires proximal motor control.
Donning hat	Requires proximal strength and grip strength.

5. Task: Zipping jacket

Key Impairments Addressed:
1. Decreased proximal strength
2. Decreased distal strength
3. Decreased pinch grip
4. Decreased distal motor control

Materials:
Jacket with zipper

Task Description:
1. Grasp zipper with affected hand.
2. Zip jacket, then unzip and release zipper.

Grading Task:

Increase difficulty	Decrease difficulty
Use a jacket with a small zipper. • Requires more distal motor control.	Use a jacket with a large zipper. • Requires less distal motor control.
Wear a jacket or place it on a hanger to zip. • Requires more proximal strength.	Place a jacket on a table or lap to zip. • Requires less proximal strength.

Task Mastery:
1. Grasps and pulls zipper on first attempt.

Ideas for related tasks	Rationale
Sealing a resealable bag	Requires pinch grip. Requires distal motor control.
Zipping a purse	Requires pinch grip. Requires distal motor control.

6. Task: Folding socks

Key Impairments Addressed:
1. Decreased distal strength
2. Decreased grip strength
3. Decreased distal motor control

Materials:
Socks of various sizes

Task Description:
1. Grasp socks with bilateral hands and fold together.
2. Place in basket or drawer.

Grading Task:

Increase difficulty	Decrease difficulty
Use long socks that require more folding.	Use small socks.
• Requires more distal strength and motor control.	• Requires less distal strength and motor control.

Task Mastery:
1. Consistently grasps both socks and folds on first attempt.

Ideas for related tasks	Rationale
Folding gloves	Requires distal strength and grip strength.
	Requires distal motor control.

7. Task: Brushing teeth

Key Impairments Addressed:
1. Decreased proximal strength
2. Decreased grip strength
3. Decreased distal motor control

Materials:
Toothbrush

Task Description:
1. Grasp toothbrush with affected hand.
2. Simulate brushing teeth back and forth, side to side, or up and down four times.
3. Replace toothbrush on the table.

Grading Task:

Increase difficulty	Decrease difficulty
Use standard-sized or smaller toothbrush. • Requires more grip strength.	Use a toothbrush with large handle. • Requires less grip strength.
Reach for toothbrush on shelf of medicine cabinet or in toothbrush holder. • Requires proximal strength. • Requires more proximal and distal motor control.	Place toothbrush in affected hand using unaffected hand. • Requires less proximal strength and grip strength. • Requires less proximal and distal motor control.

Task Mastery:
1. Consistently grasps toothbrush on first attempt.
2. Grasps toothbrush with effective grip type on first attempt.

Ideas for related tasks	Rationale
Shaving	Requires proximal strength and grip strength. Requires distal motor control.
Putting on lip balm	Requires grip strength. Requires distal motor control.

8. Task: Eating soup

Key Impairments Addressed:
1. Decreased distal strength
2. Decreased grip strength
3. Decreased distal motor control

Materials:
Bowl of liquid
Spoon

Task Description:
1. Grasp spoon placed on table with affected arm.
2. Scoop soup (or rice or water to simulate soup) and bring toward mouth.
3. Pour soup off of spoon back into the bowl and return spoon to table.

Grading Task:

Increase difficulty	Decrease difficulty
Use standard-sized or smaller spoon. • Requires more grip strength.	Use spoon with built-up handle. • Requires less grip strength.
Place thin liquid, such as water, into bowl. • Requires more distal motor control.	Use viscous liquid or thick soup. • Requires less distal motor control.
Use a large, deep bowl. • Requires more distal strength and motor control.	Use a small, shallow bowl. • Requires more distal strength and motor control.

Task Mastery:
1. Consistently grasps spoon with effective grip and brings to mouth on first attempt.
2. Does not drop spoon.

Ideas for related tasks	Rationale
Eating cereal	Requires distal strength and grip strength. Requires distal motor control.

9. Task: Donning and doffing jacket

Key Impairments Addressed:
1. Decreased proximal strength
2. Decreased grip strength
3. Decreased proximal motor control

Materials:
Jacket

Task Description:
1. Grasp jacket with unaffected hand and place affected arm through sleeve, then other arm through the other sleeve.
2. Doff jacket, set on table with affected hand, and repeat.

Grading Task:

Increase difficulty	Decrease difficulty
Don and doff a button-up shirt. • Requires more proximal strength and motor control.	Don and doff a vest. • Requires less proximal strength and motor control.
Grasp jacket with affected hand and don onto unaffected arm first. • Requires more proximal strength and grip strength.	Don jacket onto only affected arm without donning onto unaffected arm. • Requires less proximal strength. • Requires no grip strength.

Task Mastery:
1. Consistently demonstrates appropriate grading of arm elevation and extension for moving arm into and out of sleeve.

Ideas for related tasks	Rationale
Washing unaffected arm with affected hand	Requires proximal strength and grip strength. Requires proximal motor control.
Tucking shirt into back of pants.	Requires proximal and distal strength.

10. Task: Drinking from cup

Key Impairments Addressed:
1. Decreased proximal strength
2. Decreased distal strength
3. Decreased grip strength
4. Decreased proximal motor control

Materials:
Cups of various sizes (plastic or paper recommended, not glass)

Task Description:
1. Grasp cup with affected hand and simulate pouring into mouth.
2. Set down, release grip, and repeat.

Grading Task:

Increase difficulty	Decrease difficulty
Use a small, lightweight cup. • Requires more distal strength to achieve grasp around cup without cup tipping over or sliding.	Use a large, heavy cup. • Requires less distal strength to achieve grasp around cup because it will not slide or tip as easily.
Note. Could decrease difficulty if grip strength is more impaired than finger extension.	*Note.* Could increase difficulty if grip strength and shoulder and elbow flexion strength are more impaired than finger extension, making lifting the glass difficult.
Stand with cup on overhead shelf between grasps. • Requires more proximal strength and motor control.	Sit and place cup on table between grasps. • Requires less proximal strength and motor control.

Task Mastery:
1. Consistently grasps cup with effective grip and brings to mouth on first attempt.
2. Does not drop cup.

Ideas for related tasks	Rationale
Pouring beverage from pitcher	Requires distal strength and grip strength. Requires proximal and distal motor control.
Eating soup	Requires grip strength. Requires proximal motor control.

11. Task: Applying bandage

Key Impairments Addressed:
1. Decreased pinch grip
2. Decreased fine motor control

Materials:
Bandages of various sizes

Task Description:
1. Grasp bandage with affected hand and apply to target on body using bilateral hands.

Grading Task:

Increase difficulty	Decrease difficulty
Use small bandage with small surface area. • Requires more fine motor control.	Use bandage with larger surface area. • Requires less fine motor control.
Apply bandage to leg or opposite arm. • Requires proximal strength to reach limb.	Apply bandage to spot right in front of client. • Requires less proximal strength for reaching.
Remove bandage from paper wrapper before applying. • Requires more fine motor control.	

Task Mastery:
1. Consistently applies bandage on desired spot on first attempt.

Ideas for related tasks	Rationale
Applying a sticky note to paper	Requires pinch grip. Requires fine motor control.
Opening a resealable bag	Requires pinch grip. Requires fine motor control.

12. Task: Unwrapping piece of candy

Key Impairments Addressed:
1. Decreased pinch grip
2. Decreased fine motor control

Materials:
Pieces of candy in wrappers

Task Description:
1. Grasp candy with affected hand and use bilateral hands to open wrapper.

Grading Task:

Increase difficulty	Decrease difficulty
Unwrap small pieces of candy.	Unwrap large pieces of candy.
• Requires more fine motor control.	• Requires less fine motor control.
Unwrap candy with various types of wrappers.	Unwrap same type of candy.
• Requires more fine motor control.	• Requires less fine motor control.

Task Mastery:
1. Consistently unwraps each piece of candy on first attempt.

Ideas for related tasks	Rationale
Unwrapping a slice of cheese	Requires pinch grip. Requires fine motor control.
Unwrapping a piece of gum	Requires pinch grip. Requires fine motor control.
Opening a bandage	Requires pinch grip. Requires fine motor control.

13. Task: Grasping shoes from shoebox

Key Impairments Addressed:
1. Decreased proximal strength
2. Decreased grip strength

Materials:
Shoebox
Shoes

Task Description:
1. Open shoe box with affected hand while unaffected hand stabilizes.
2. Pull shoes out of box with affected hand.

Grading Task:

Increase difficulty	Decrease difficulty
Use heavy shoes.	Use lightweight shoes or sandals.
• Requires more proximal strength and grip strength.	• Requires less proximal strength and grip strength.
Use shoebox with tight-fitting lid.	Use shoebox with loose-fitting lid.
• Requires more proximal strength and grip strength.	• Requires less proximal strength and grip strength.

Task Mastery:
1. Consistently opens box on first attempt.
2. Grasps shoes without dropping on first attempt.

Ideas for related tasks	Rationale
Unpacking boxes	Requires proximal strength and grip strength.
Packing and unpacking backpack	Requires proximal strength and grip strength.

14. Task: Filing fingernails

Key Impairments Addressed:
1. Decreased pinch grip
2. Decreased distal motor control

Materials:
Emery board

Task Description:
1. Grasp emery board with affected hand.
2. Simulate filing nail of opposite hand for three to four strokes.
3. Set board down and repeat for next nail.

Grading Task:

Increase difficulty	Decrease difficulty
Use a small emery board.	Use a large emery board.
• Requires more distal motor control.	• Requires less distal motor control.

Task Mastery:
1. Consistently grasps emery board on first attempt.
2. Demonstrates smooth, coordinated motion during filing.
3. Does not drop board.

Ideas for related tasks	Rationale
Clipping fingernails	Requires pinch grip. Requires fine motor control.
Applying polish to fingernails	Requires pinch grip. Requires fine motor control.

15. Task: Donning and doffing socks

Key Impairments Addressed:
1. Decreased distal strength
2. Decreased grip strength
3. Decreased distal motor control

Materials:
Socks

Task Description:
1. Grasp sock.
2. Don one at a time with bilateral hands.
3. Doff one at a time and repeat.

Grading Task:

Increase difficulty	Decrease difficulty
Use tall socks with tight-fitting elastic.	Use short, loose socks.
• Requires more grip strength.	• Requires less grip strength.

Task Mastery:
1. Consistently grasps socks on first attempt.
2. Dons and doffs on first attempt.

Ideas for related tasks	Rationale
Donning and doffing shoes	Requires distal strength. Requires distal motor control.
Donning and doffing ankle–foot orthosis	Requires distal strength. Requires distal motor control.
Donning and doffing pants	Requires proximal and distal strength.

16. Task: Opening and closing umbrella

Key Impairments Addressed:
1. Decreased proximal strength
2. Decreased pinch grip

Materials:
Umbrella

Task Description:
1. Hold umbrella handle with unaffected hand.
2. Press button and push umbrella open with affected hand.
3. Pull umbrella closed with affected hand.

Grading Task:

Increase difficulty	Decrease difficulty
Use a large, heavy umbrella.	Use a small, lightweight umbrella.
• Requires more proximal strength to open and close umbrella.	• Requires less proximal strength.
Use umbrella cover, removing with affected hand.	
• Requires more grip strength.	

Task Mastery:
1. Consistently opens and closes umbrella on first attempt.

Idea for related task	Rationale
Opening and closing window blinds	Requires pinch grip to grasp string or chain.
	Requires proximal motor control to pull down or up.

17. Task: Pumping soap from dispenser

Key Impairments Addressed:
1. Decreased proximal strength
2. Decreased proximal motor control

Materials:
Soap dispenser

Task Description:
1. Reach for soap dispenser.
2. Pump soap.
3. Return arm to side and repeat.

Grading Task:

Increase difficulty	Decrease difficulty
Use a dispenser that is stiff when pumping.	Use a dispenser that is easy to pump.
• Requires more proximal strength.	• Requires less proximal strength.
Place dispenser at arm's length from client.	Place dispenser close to client.
• Requires more proximal strength and motor control.	• Requires less proximal strength and motor control.

Task Mastery:
1. Consistently pumps out soap on first attempt.
2. Does not tip over soap dispenser.

Ideas for related tasks	Rationale
Pumping ketchup dispenser	Requires proximal strength and motor control.
Pumping lotion	Requires proximal strength and motor control.

18. Task: Washing hair

Key Impairments Addressed:
1. Decreased proximal strength
2. Decreased distal strength
3. Decreased proximal motor control

Materials:
Shampoo bottle

Task Description:
1. Grasp bottle with affected hand and pour shampoo into unaffected hand.
2. Rub hands together and wash (or simulate washing) hair.

Grading Task:

Increase difficulty	Decrease difficulty
Wash all over head.	Wash only the front of the head.
• Requires more proximal strength and motor control.	• Requires less proximal strength and motor control.

Task Mastery:
1. Consistently grasps and pours shampoo out on first attempt.
2. Does not drop bottle.
3. Demonstrates smooth, coordinated motion during washing.

Ideas for related tasks	Rationale
Washing body	Requires proximal strength and grip strength. Requires proximal motor control.
Styling hair	Requires proximal strength and grip strength. Requires proximal motor control.
Drying hair	Requires proximal strength and grip strength. Requires proximal motor control.
Brushing hair	Requires proximal strength and grip strength. Requires proximal motor control.

19. Task: Donning and doffing eyeglasses

Key Impairments Addressed:
1. Decreased distal strength
2. Decreased grip strength
3. Decreased distal motor control

Materials:
Eyeglasses or sunglasses

Task Description:
1. Grasp eyeglasses with affected hand.
2. Use bilateral hands to unfold stems and don.

Grading Task:

Increase difficulty	Decrease difficulty
Use glasses with thin stems.	Use glasses with thick stems.
• Requires more distal motor control.	• Requires less distal motor control.
Fold stems of glasses after doffing.	Leave stems unfolded between doffing and donning.
• Requires more distal motor control.	• Requires less distal motor control.

Task Mastery:
1. Consistently dons and doffs glasses on first attempt.
2. Does not drop glasses.

Idea for related task	Rationale
Donning and doffing hat	Requires proximal strength and grip strength.

20. Task: Donning wristwatch

Key Impairments Addressed:
1. Decreased grip strength
2. Decreased distal motor control

Materials:
Wristwatch

Task Description:
1. Grasp wristwatch with affected hand and don on opposite wrist.
2. Remove from wrist and set on table.

Grading Task:

Increase difficulty	Decrease difficulty
Don and doff a small wristwatch.	Don and doff a large wristwatch.
• Requires more fine motor control.	• Requires less fine motor control.
Don and doff wristwatch with clasp.	Don and doff wristwatch with elastic band.
• Requires more distal motor control.	• Requires less distal motor control.

Task Mastery:
1. Consistently grasps and releases watch on first attempt.
2. Dons and doffs without dropping.

Idea for related task	Rationale
Donning a bracelet	Requires grip strength.
	Requires distal motor control.

21. Task: Shaving face

Key Impairments Addressed:
1. Decreased distal strength
2. Decreased pinch grip
3. Decreased distal motor control

Materials:
Razor (manual or electric) with cap left on

Task Description:
1. Grasp shaving cream and simulate squeezing out of can with affected hand.
2. Use bilateral hands to simulate rubbing on face.
3. Grasp razor with affected hand and simulate shaving three to four strokes.
4. Rinse razor off under water, then set razor down and repeat Steps 3 and 4.

Grading Task:

Increase difficulty	Decrease difficulty
Stand up and set razor in small cup on shelf between sets. • Requires more proximal strength and motor control.	Sit down and set razor on table between sets. • Requires less proximal strength and motor control.
Use small razor. • Requires more grip strength. • Requires more fine motor control.	Use razor with adapted handle or electric razor. • Requires less grip strength. • Requires less fine motor control.

Task Mastery:
1. Grasps and releases razor on first attempt.
2. Shaving strokes are coordinated, with smooth movement trajectory.

Ideas for related tasks	Rationale
Applying makeup	Requires distal strength and motor control.
Shaving underarms or legs	Requires distal strength. Requires proximal and distal motor control.

22. Task: Applying deodorant

Key Impairments Addressed:
1. Decreased proximal strength
2. Decreased distal strength

Materials:
Deodorant

Task Description:
1. Grasp deodorant with affected hand.
2. Apply under arm or simulate application.
3. Set deodorant down on table and repeat.

Grading Task:

Increase difficulty	Decrease difficulty
Use wide deodorant bottle. • Requires more distal strength to grasp bottle.	Use narrow deodorant bottle. • Requires less distal strength to grasp bottle.
Note. May decrease the difficulty level depending on hand impairments.	*Note.* May increase the difficulty level depending on hand impairments.
Remove cap with affected hand. • Requires more grip strength.	Remove cap with unaffected hand. • Requires less grip strength.

Task Mastery:
1. Consistently grasps bottle and reaches target on first attempt.
2. Does not tip or drop bottle.

Ideas for related tasks	Rationale
Washing underarm	Requires proximal strength and grip strength.
Shaving underarm	Requires proximal strength and distal strength. Requires distal motor control.

23. Task: Donning and doffing gloves

Key Impairments Addressed:
1. Decreased distal strength
2. Decreased distal motor control

Materials:
Gloves

Task Description:
1. Grasp glove with affected hand and don onto unaffected hand.
2. Grasp glove with unaffected hand and don onto affected hand.

Grading Task:

Increase difficulty	Decrease difficulty
Use small gloves.	Use mittens or oversized gloves.
• Requires more distal strength and motor control.	• Requires less distal strength and motor control.
Retrieve gloves from coat pocket while standing.	Pick glove up from table while sitting.
• Requires more distal strength and motor control.	• Requires less distal strength and motor control.

Task Mastery:
1. Consistently dons and doffs bilateral gloves on first attempt.
2. Does not drop glove.

Ideas for related tasks	Rationale
Donning and doffing a jacket	Requires proximal and distal strength.
	Requires grip strength.
	Requires proximal motor control.
Applying hand lotion	Requires distal strength.

Exhibit 4.4. Productivity Tasks

24. Task: Typing

Key Impairments Addressed:
1. Decreased distal strength
2. Decreased fine motor control

Materials:
Computer monitor and keyboard or laptop
Computer typing program or paper from which to copy words

Task Description:
1. Type words from computer typing program or copy words from paper.
2. Use bilateral hands.

Grading Task:

Increase difficulty	Decrease difficulty
Type long words. • Requires more fine motor control.	Type shorter words. • Requires less fine motor control.
Increase speed at which client must type. • Requires more fine motor control.	Type at self-selected pace. • Requires less fine motor control.
Type on small keyboard or laptop. • Requires more fine motor control.	Type on large keyboard. • Requires less fine motor control.

Task Mastery:
1. Consistently types the correct letters with minimal errors.
2. Consistently uses affected hand for appropriate letters on the basis of keyboard location.

Ideas for related tasks	Rationale
Dialing phone numbers on telephone	Requires fine motor control.
Pressing buttons on cell phone	Requires fine motor control.

25. Task: Handwriting

Key Impairments Addressed:
1. Decreased pinch grip
2. Decreased fine motor control

Materials:
Ink pen or pencil
Paper
Article or template from which to copy words

Task Description:
1. Sit with materials on table.
2. Grasp ink pen and copy words from article or template.

Grading Task:

Increase difficulty	Decrease difficulty
Use small ink pen. • Requires more fine motor control.	Use large pen or pen with built-up body. • Requires less fine motor control.
Write on lined paper. • Requires more fine motor control.	Write on blank printer paper. • Requires less fine motor control.
Copy long words or words from news article. • Requires more fine motor control.	Write signature or short words. • Requires less fine motor control.
Write on chalkboard or dry-erase board. • Requires more proximal and distal motor control.	Initialing or check-marking legal forms. • Requires less proximal and distal motor control.

Task Mastery:
1. Consistently writes on the lines.
2. Does not drop writing tool.
3. Reaches goal for quality or speed of handwriting.

Ideas for related tasks	Rationale
Drawing	Requires fine motor control. Requires pinch grip.
Cutting with utility knife	Requires grip strength.
Sorting pills	Requires fine motor control. Requires pinch grip.

26. Task: Clicking computer mouse

Key Impairments Addressed:
1. Decreased distal strength
2. Decreased fine motor control

Materials:
Computer screen with mouse or laptop with touchpad

Task Description:
1. Sit with computer screen with mouse or laptop with touchpad on table.
2. Place affected hand on mouse or touchpad and play computer game or navigate icons.

Grading Task:

Increase difficulty	Decrease difficulty
Choose game or icons requiring small targets to click, or click and drag to a target. • Requires more fine motor control.	Choose large targets. • Requires less fine motor control.
Select targets spaced widely apart. • Requires more fine motor control and distal strength.	Select targets spaced closely together. • Requires less fine motor control and distal strength.
Use laser mouse or change precision to increase sensitivity to movement. • Requires more fine motor control.	Use ball mouse or change precision of mouse to decrease sensitivity to movement. • Requires less fine motor control.

Task Mastery:
1. Consistently places hand on mouse or touchpad effectively on first attempt.
2. Consistently selects target on first attempt.

Ideas for related tasks	Rationale
Navigating electronic reader or tablet	Requires fine motor control.
Typing text message on cell phone	Requires fine motor control.

27. Task: Counting money

Key Impairments Addressed:
1. Decreased pinch grip
2. Decreased fine motor control

Materials:
Play money
Change

Task Description:
1. Sit with stack of bills in unaffected hand.
2. Count out bills one at a time with affected hand and hand to practitioner.

   or

1. Place coins in affected palm.
2. Transfer coins to fingertips, and hand them to practitioner.

Grading Task:

Increase difficulty	Decrease difficulty
Place bills in wallet or coins in coin pouch. • Requires more fine motor control and distal strength.	Place bills or coins on table. • Requires less fine motor control and distal strength.
Select only one type of coin from pile of various coins. • Requires more fine motor control.	Place coins in unaffected palm, and select coin with fingers of affected hand. • Requires less fine motor control.
Place coins in coin bank. • Requires more proximal and distal motor control.	Place coins in side pocket of pants. • Requires less proximal and distal motor control.

Task Mastery:
1. Consistently grasps correct bill or coin on first attempt.
2. Consistently reaches target in which to place bill or coin.

Ideas for related tasks	Rationale
Sorting pills	Requires pinch grip. Requires fine motor control.
Sorting mail	Requires pinch grip. Requires proximal and distal motor control.
Turning pages	Requires pinch grip. Requires fine motor control.

28. Task: Organizing toolbox

Key Impairments Addressed:
1. Decreased proximal strength
2. Decreased grip strength
3. Decreased proximal motor control

Materials:
Toolbox with tools

Task Description:
1. Grasp tool, remove from toolbox, and place on table; repeat for all tools.
2. Place each tool back into toolbox.

Grading Task:

Increase difficulty	Decrease difficulty
Grasp large tools of various shapes. • Requires more distal strength.	Grasp small tools of similar shapes. • Requires less distal strength.
Grasp heavy tools (i.e., hammer). • Requires more proximal strength and grip strength.	Grasp lightweight tools. • Requires less proximal strength and grip strength.
Position toolbox at more distance from client or elevated on shelf. • Requires more proximal strength.	Position toolbox close to client. • Requires less proximal strength.

Task Mastery:
1. Consistently grasps tool and places into or out of box on first attempt.
2. Demonstrates smooth trajectory of motion during reach.

Ideas for related tasks	Rationale
Organizing tackle box	Requires proximal strength and motor control.
Cleaning out drawer	Requires proximal and grip strength. Requires proximal motor control.

29. Task: Navigating digital tablet or e-reader

Key Impairments Addressed:
1. Decreased distal strength
2. Decreased fine motor control

Materials:
Digital tablet or e-reader
Program or keypad requiring tapping or swiping motion

Task Description:
1. With tablet on tabletop or lap, navigate by tapping icon or swiping screen.

Grading Task:

Increase difficulty	Decrease difficulty
Use small device. • Requires more fine motor control to select target.	Use large device. • Requires less fine motor control to select target.
Select small target to tap. • Requires more fine motor control.	Tap large target or turn page with swiping motion. • Requires less fine motor control.
Place device on angle or hold in unaffected upper extremity. • Requires more proximal strength and fine motor control.	

Task Mastery:
1. Consistently taps correct target on first attempt.
2. Demonstrates smooth trajectory of movement during swiping.

Ideas for related tasks	Rationale
Using remote control	Requires proximal and distal motor control.
Dialing a phone	Requires fine motor control.
Dealing playing cards	Requires proximal and fine motor control.
Clicking computer mouse	Requires fine motor control.

30. Task: Sewing

Key Impairments Addressed:
1. Decreased distal strength
2. Decreased pinch grip
3. Decreased fine motor control

Materials:
Sewing needle (plastic, blunt-tipped needle suggested for safety)
Thread
Cloth (or other material through which to push sewing needle)

Task Description:
1. Grasp threaded needle.
2. Push needle through cloth; adjust grip and pull thread through.

Grading Task:

Increase difficulty	Decrease difficulty
Use firm material through which it may be difficult to push the needle. • Requires more grip strength.	Use thin material. • Requires less grip strength.
Use small needle. • Requires more fine motor control.	Use large needle. • Requires less fine motor control.

Task Mastery:
1. Does not drop needle.
2. Consistently grasps and pushes needle through material on first attempt.

Ideas for related tasks	Rationale
Weaving a basket	Requires fine motor control. Requires pinch grip.
Using a latch hook	Requires fine motor control. Requires pinch grip.

31. Task: Flipping light switch

Key Impairments Addressed:
1. Decreased proximal strength
2. Decreased pinch grip
3. Decreased proximal motor control

Materials:
Light switch

Task Description:
1. Stand near doorway and flip light switch on and off with affected upper extremity.

Grading Task:

Increase difficulty	Decrease difficulty
Stand further away from switch.	Stand next to switch.
• Requires more proximal strength and motor control.	• Requires less proximal strength and motor control.
Use dimmer dial.	Use standard light switch.
• Requires more fine motor control.	• Requires less fine motor control.
Pull string on overhead light bulb.	
• Requires more proximal strength and motor control.	

Task Mastery:
1. Consistently flips light switch on first attempt.
2. Demonstrates smooth trajectory of movement during reach.

Ideas for related tasks	Rationale
Folding down sun visor in car	Requires proximal strength and motor control.
Pulling shades down	Requires proximal strength and motor control.

32. Task: Cutting food

Key Impairments Addressed:
1. Decreased proximal strength
2. Decreased grip strength
3. Decreased proximal motor control
4. Decreased distal motor control

Materials:
Silverware

Food (hand exercise putty, play dough, or other nonperishable material recommended)

Task Description:
1. Grasp silverware.
2. Press fork into food to stabilize food.
3. Cut food with knife.
4. Set silverware down on tabletop.

Note. This is an example of a task in which the affected hand could be trained as the stabilizing hand or the cutting hand, depending on the eventual goal.

Grading Task:

Increase difficulty	Decrease difficulty
Use small knife or fork. • Requires more distal strength and motor control.	Use adapted knife or fork with built-up handle. • Requires less distal strength and motor control.
Press or cut into firm material. • Requires more grip strength.	Press or cut into soft material. • Requires less grip strength.
Place multiple items of food on plate. • Requires more proximal and distal motor control.	Place one large food item on large plate. • Requires less proximal and distal motor control.
Set paper plate with food on a smooth table on which it may slide more readily. • Requires more distal strength and motor control.	Set food on plate with nonslip material underneath it. • Requires less distal strength and motor control.

Task Mastery:
1. Consistently grasps and releases silverware on first attempt.
2. Demonstrates coordinated movement during cutting.

Ideas for related tasks	Rationale
Opening envelope with letter opener	Requires distal strength. Requires proximal and distal motor control.
Cutting boxes with utility knife	Requires distal strength. Requires proximal and distal motor control.

33. Task: Removing lids

Key Impairments Addressed:

1. Decreased distal strength
2. Decreased grip strength
3. Decreased distal motor control

Materials:

Containers (a variety of different containers with different lids, flip tops or screw tops, recommended)

Task Description:

1. Grasp container with unaffected hand.
2. Remove lid with affected hand.
3. Replace lid with affected hand.

Note. This is an example of a task in which the affected hand could be trained as the stabilizing hand or the removing hand, depending on the eventual goal.

Grading Task:

Increase difficulty	Decrease difficulty
Select containers with wide lids. • Requires more distal strength and motor control.	Select containers with small lids. • Requires less distal strength and motor control.
Tighten lids before client removes or select lids that are more difficult to remove. • Requires more distal strength.	Loosen lids before client removes. • Requires less distal strength.
Use containers with twist lids. • Requires more distal motor control.	Use lids that pop off or flip open. • Requires less distal motor control.

Task Mastery:

1. Consistently removes and replaces lid on first attempt.
2. Demonstrates smooth movement while removing or twisting open lids.

Ideas for related tasks	Rationale
Turning faucet	Requires distal strength and motor control.
Turning doorknob	Requires distal strength and motor control.

34. Task: Removing towels from laundry basket

Key Impairments Addressed:
1. Decreased proximal strength
2. Decreased grip strength

Materials:
Towels
Laundry basket

Task Description:
1. Stand at table with laundry basket of towels on table top.
2. Grasp towel, lift it from basket with affected hand, and place on table.
3. Release grip and continue with remaining towels.
4. Place each towel back into basket.

Grading Task:

Increase difficulty	Decrease difficulty
Use large bath towels or bed sheets. • Requires more proximal and distal strength.	Use washcloths or hand towels. • Requires less proximal and distal strength.
Place towels in deep basket. • Requires more proximal strength.	Use shallow basket, or place towels in pile on table. • Requires less proximal strength.
Incorporate lifting laundry basket from table to a chair or floor. • Requires more proximal and grip strength.	Sit down, with basket on floor in front of or next to client. • Requires less postural control so client can focus on upper-extremity movement.

Task Mastery:
1. Consistently grasps and releases towels without dropping.
2. Consistently reaches target in which to place towels (i.e., laundry basket or table top).

Ideas for related tasks	Rationale
Pulling clothes out of dryer	Requires upper extremity extension and grip strength.
Unloading groceries from grocery bag	Requires shoulder elevation and elbow extension to reach into and out of bag.

35. Task: Folding towels

Key Impairments Addressed:
1. Decreased proximal strength
2. Decreased grip strength
3. Decreased distal motor control

Materials:
Towels
Laundry basket (optional)

Task Description:
1. Stand at table with towels in pile.
2. Grasp towels one at a time with affected upper extremity and fold into fourths using bilateral upper extremities.
3. Stack towels.

Grading Task:

Increase difficulty	Decrease difficulty
Use large linens, such as bath towels or sheets. • Requires more proximal strength and grip strength.	Use small washcloths or hand towels. • Requires less proximal strength and grip strength.
Stack folded linens on shelf. • Requires more proximal strength.	Place each folded linen onto table top. • Requires less proximal strength.
Fold towels while standing and holding them up in air. • Requires more proximal strength and grip strength.	Fold towels on table top while sitting down. • Requires less proximal strength. • More attention can be focused on upper-extremity movements.

Task Mastery:
1. Consistently meets opposite corners with each fold.
2. Consistently grasps and releases linens on first attempt.

Ideas for related tasks	Rationale
Folding clothes	Requires proximal strength and grip strength.
Hanging clothes on hanger	Requires proximal strength and grip strength.

36. Task: Hanging clothes on hangers

Key Impairments Addressed:
1. Decreased proximal strength
2. Decreased grip strength
3. Decreased proximal motor control
4. Decreased distal motor control

Materials:
Hangers
Shirts
Coat rack or hook

Task Description:
1. Grasp shirt from table or back of a chair using affected hand.
2. Use bilateral hands to place shirt on hanger.
3. Use affected upper extremity to hang shirt on rack or hook.

Grading Task:

Increase difficulty	Decrease difficulty
Use heavy sweater or coat. • Requires more proximal strength and grip strength.	Use t-shirt or blouse. • Requires less proximal strength and grip strength.
Use hook or coat rack that is elevated overhead. • Requires more proximal strength and motor control.	Use hook or coat rack that is lower to ground. • Requires less proximal strength and motor control.
Use plastic hanger that requires more precise placement because shirt slips off. • Requires more distal motor control.	Use hanger with rubber ends that holds shirt in place. • Requires less distal motor control.

Task Mastery:
1. Does not drop shirt or hanger.
2. Consistently places shirt on hanger on first attempt.

Idea for related task	Rationale
Hanging clothes on clothesline	Requires proximal strength and grip strength. Requires proximal motor control.

37. Task: Placing cans on shelf

Key Impairments Addressed:
1. Decreased proximal strength
2. Decreased grip strength
3. Decreased proximal motor control

Materials:
Cans
Cabinet

Task Description:
1. Stand at cabinet.
2. Grasp can from table top and place in cabinet.
3. Repeat for multiple cans, return can to table top, or both.

Grading Task:

Increase difficulty	Decrease difficulty
Lift cans to high shelf. • Requires more proximal strength.	Lift cans to low shelf. • Requires less proximal strength.
Lift heavy cans or wide cans. • Requires more proximal and distal strength.	Stack lightweight or small cans. • Requires less proximal and distal strength.
Remove cans from simulated dishwasher or low cabinet before placing on shelf. • Requires more proximal motor control.	

Task Mastery:
1. Consistently grasps and releases can on first attempt.
2. Does not drop can.
3. Demonstrates smooth trajectory of movement.

Ideas for related tasks	Rationale
Removing books from bookshelf	Requires proximal strength and grip strength. Requires proximal motor control.
Retrieving bottle from refrigerator	Requires proximal strength and grip strength. Requires proximal motor control.
Unloading or loading dishwasher	Requires proximal strength and grip strength. Requires proximal motor control.

38. Task: Sweeping floor

Key Impairments Addressed:
1. Decreased proximal strength
2. Decreased grip strength
3. Decreased distal motor control

Materials:
Broom
Dustpan
Scraps of paper

Task Description:
1. Grasp broom and sweep scraps of paper into a pile.
2. Sweep paper into dustpan.
3. Place paper back on floor and repeat.

Grading Task:

Increase difficulty	Decrease difficulty
Sweep paper a longer distance away or walk around room and sweep it into several piles. • Requires more proximal strength.	Sweep paper a short distance. • Requires less proximal strength.
Sweep many small pieces of paper into pile. • Requires more distal motor control.	Sweep a few large scraps of paper. • Requires less distal motor control.

Task Mastery:
1. Consistently demonstrates appropriate grip on broom.
2. Consistently sweeps all paper into a pile in few attempts.

Ideas for related tasks	Rationale
Vacuuming	Requires proximal strength and grip strength.
Shoveling	Requires proximal strength and grip strength.

39. Task: Opening door

Key Impairments Addressed:
1. Decreased proximal strength
2. Decreased distal strength
3. Decreased distal motor control

Materials:
Door with doorknob

Note. Choose round or horizontal handle on the basis of the client's impairments and what type of doorknobs client has at home.

Task Description:
1. Stand at door.
2. Grasp knob and turn to open.
3. Release knob, grasp knob again, and pull door closed.

Grading Task:

Increase difficulty	Decrease difficulty
Select large doorknob.	Select small doorknob.
• Requires more distal strength.	• Requires less distal strength.
Select stiff doorknob.	Select loose doorknob.
• Requires more distal strength.	• Requires less distal strength.

Task Mastery:
1. Consistently grasps and turns doorknob on first attempt.
2. Consistently demonstrates appropriate timing of finger movement around knob to grasp and release.

Ideas for related tasks	Rationale
Turning on garden hose	Requires distal strength.
Turning on sink faucet	Requires distal strength.
Opening cabinet	Requires proximal and distal strength.

40. Task: Drying pots and pans

Key Impairments Addressed:
1. Decreased proximal strength
2. Decreased grip strength
3. Decreased proximal motor control

Materials:
Pots and pans
Towel
Drying rack

Task Description:
1. Grasp pot with unaffected hand.
2. Grasp towel with affected hand and simulate drying with three strokes.
3. Release towel.

Grading Task:

Increase difficulty	Decrease difficulty
Switch hands and grasp pot with affected hand, drying with unaffected hand. • Requires more proximal strength and grip strength.	Dry with small washcloth in affected hand. • Requires less proximal strength and grip strength.
Dry large pot or pan. • Requires more grip strength.	Dry small bowl or plate. • Requires less grip strength.

Task Mastery:
1. Consistently grasps and releases towel on first attempt.
2. Demonstrates smooth trajectory of movement during drying.

Ideas for related tasks	Rationale
Wiping countertop	Requires proximal strength and motor control.
Dusting	Requires proximal strength and motor control.

41. Task: Sanding wall

Key Impairments Addressed:
1. Decreased proximal strength
2. Decreased grip strength
3. Decreased proximal motor control

Materials:
Hand sander
Wall
Optional: targets on wall

Task Description:
1. Grasp hand sander and lift from table.
2. Sand wall, moving back and forth between targets, three to four times.
3. Set sander down on table.

Grading Task:

Increase difficulty	Decrease difficulty
Increase distance between targets. • Requires more proximal strength and motor control.	Decrease distance between targets. • Requires less proximal strength and motor control.
Vary the motions required for sanding (i.e., abduction–adduction vs. flexion–extension vs. counterclockwise–clockwise). • Requires more proximal strength and motor control.	Consistently sand with same motion. • Requires less proximal strength and motor control.
Stand up and move to various spots on wall or ceiling to sand. • Requires more proximal strength and motor control.	Sit down and sand object at table. • Requires less proximal strength and motor control. • More attention can be focused on task.

Task Mastery:
1. Consistently grasps sander on first attempt.
2. Demonstrates smooth motions during sanding.

Ideas for related tasks	Rationale
Washing windows	Requires proximal strength and motor control.
Dusting tables	Requires proximal strength and motor control.

42. Task: Sorting silverware

Key Impairments Addressed:
1. Decreased grip strength
2. Decreased fine motor control

Materials:
Silverware
Drawer organizer

Task Description:
1. Use affected hand to grasp one item from pile of silverware on the table and place it in designated slot of drawer organizer.
2. Release item into slot.

Grading Task:

Increase difficulty	Decrease difficulty
Stand and reach down for silverware before placing in drawer to simulate unloading silverware from dishwasher. • Requires more proximal motor control.	Place silverware on table in front of client. • Requires less proximal motor control.
Use thin silverware or plastic ware. • Requires more fine motor control.	Use large utensils, such as spatulas or ladles, and place in drawer without organizer. • Requires less fine motor control.
Select one type of utensil from pile of various types (i.e., fork from pile of spoons, knives, and forks). • Requires more fine motor control to sort through utensils.	Place only one type of utensil on the table to grasp and place into organizer. • Requires less fine motor control.

Task Mastery:
1. Consistently selects appropriate utensil and places into designated spot of organizer on first attempt.
2. Does not drop silverware.

Ideas for related tasks	Rationale
Placing pencils into pencil holder	Requires grip strength. Requires fine motor control.
Setting the dinner table	Requires grip strength. Requires fine motor control.
Organizing toolbox	Requires grip strength. Requires fine motor control.

43. Task: Answering telephone

Key Impairments Addressed:
1. Decreased proximal strength
2. Decreased grip strength
3. Decreased proximal motor control

Materials:
Telephone (cellular or landline)

Task Description:
1. Stand at counter.
2. Pick phone up from countertop or from receiver with affected hand and bring to ear.
3. Return phone to countertop or receiver.

Grading Task:

Increase difficulty	Decrease difficulty
Stand with phone in purse pocket or in protective case. • Requires proximal and distal motor control.	Sit down with phone in lap or in front on table. • Requires less proximal and distal motor control.
Stand with phone on receiver against wall. • Requires proximal strength and motor control.	

Task Mastery:
1. Consistently grasps and brings telephone up to ear.
2. Does not drop phone or readjust in hand.

Idea for related task	Rationale
Picking up a hairbrush	Requires proximal strength and grip strength. Requires proximal motor control.

44. Task: Assembling nut and bolt

Key Impairments Addressed:
1. Decreased distal strength
2. Decreased pinch grip
3. Decreased fine motor control

Materials:
Nuts and bolts

Task Description:
1. Grasp bolt with unaffected hand and nut with affected hand.
2. Thread nut onto bolt for three revolutions.
3. Remove nut from bolt and set them down.

Grading Task:

Increase difficulty	Decrease difficulty
Use small nuts and bolts. • Requires more fine motor control.	Use large nuts and bolts. • Requires less fine motor control.
Fix bolt in place, then fasten nut. • Requires more distal strength and fine motor control.	Hold bolt in hand at preferred angle to fasten nut. • Requires less distal strength and less fine motor control.
Fix bolt horizontally against wall. • Requires more distal strength and fine motor control.	

Task Mastery:
1. Consistently grasps nut and bolt without dropping.
2. Twists nut onto bolt for all three revolutions without pausing.
3. Removes nut from bolt and sets down without dropping.

Ideas for related tasks	Rationale
Sewing	Requires pinch grip. Requires proximal motor control. Requires fine motor control.
Threading beads onto a cord to make a necklace	Requires pinch grip. Requires proximal motor control. Requires fine motor control.

45. Task: Driving screw into wood

Key Impairments Addressed:
1. Decreased distal strength
2. Decreased grip strength
3. Decreased distal motor control

Materials:
Screwdriver
Screws
Block of wood

Task Description:
1. Grasp screw with unaffected hand and screwdriver with affected hand.
2. Drive screw into wood, turning screwdriver three revolutions.
3. Set screwdriver down and repeat.

Grading Task:

Increase difficulty	Decrease difficulty
Use long screwdriver with narrow handle. • Requires more distal strength and motor control.	Use short screwdriver with wide handle. • Requires less distal strength and motor control.
Stand and drive screws into wall or upright piece of wood. • Requires more distal strength and motor control.	Sit at table and drive screws into block of wood flat on table. • Requires less distal strength and motor control.
Use small screws. • Requires more distal motor control for placement of screwdriver into screw.	Use large screws. • Requires less distal motor control for placement of screwdriver into screw.

Task Mastery:
1. Grasps and releases screwdriver without dropping.
2. Turns screw three revolutions without pausing.

Ideas for related tasks	Rationale
Turning faucet on and off	Requires distal strength and motor control.
Turning dial on radio	Requires distal strength and motor control.
Twisting cap off of bottle	Requires distal strength and motor control.

46. Task: Fastening paperclip to papers

Key Impairments Addressed:
1. Decreased pinch grip
2. Decreased fine motor control

Materials:
Stacks of papers
Paperclips

Task Description:
1. Grasp paperclip with affected hand and stack of papers with unaffected hand.
2. Fasten paperclip to papers, then set stack of papers down with affected hand.

Grading Task:

Increase difficulty	Decrease difficulty
Use small paperclips. • Requires more fine motor control.	Use large paperclips or binder clips. • Requires less fine motor control.
Stand during the task, and set papers in hanging folder against wall after paper clipping. • Requires proximal strength and motor control.	Sit with papers and paperclips on table, and set stack on table after assembling. • Requires less proximal strength.
Retrieve paperclips from cup or small tray. • Requires more fine motor control.	Place paperclips in pile on table. • Requires less fine motor control.

Task Mastery:
1. Consistently grasps paperclip without dropping.
2. Fastens paperclip to papers on first attempt.

Idea for related task	Rationale
Fastening binder clip to papers	Requires pinch grip. Requires fine motor control.

47. Task: Filling out forms

Key Impairments Addressed:
1. Decreased pinch grip
2. Decreased fine motor control

Materials:
Papers with blank lines for signatures, dates, and checkmarks
Pen
Clipboard (optional)

Task Description:
1. Grasp pen with affected hand and fill out forms.

Grading Task:

Increase difficulty	Decrease difficulty
Use small pen.	Use adaptive pen.
• Requires more fine motor control.	• Requires less grip strength and fine motor control.
Use paper with a small space for signing.	Use paper with a large space for signing.
• Requires more fine motor control.	• Requires less fine motor control.
Set paper on clipboard on lap.	Sit with paper on table to complete forms.
• Requires more fine motor control.	• Requires less fine motor control.

Task Mastery:
1. Consistently grasps pen on first attempt.
2. Consistently and legibly marks form on the line.

Ideas for related tasks	Rationale
Writing a check	Requires pinch grip.
	Requires fine motor control.
Handwriting	Requires pinch grip.
	Require fine motor control.

48. Task: Locking door

Key Impairments Addressed:
1. Decreased distal strength
2. Decreased grip strength
3. Decreased distal motor control

Materials:
Key
Keyhole
Lock

Task Description:
1. Grasp key with affected hand and insert into keyhole.
2. Lock and unlock the lock, and remove key.

Grading Task:

Increase difficulty	Decrease difficulty
Use small key attached to key ring containing several keys.	Use large key attached to key ring with no other keys attached.
• Requires more fine motor control.	• Requires less fine motor control.
Use stiff lock or deadbolt.	Lock large, loose deadbolt instead of using key.
• Requires more distal strength.	• Requires less distal strength.

Task Mastery:
1. Grasps key and inserts into keyhole on first attempt.
2. Does not drop key.

Ideas for related tasks	Rationale
Turning a dial	Requires pinch grip.
	Requires distal motor control.
Setting a timer	Requires pinch grip.
	Requires distal motor control.

49. Task: Placing coins into vending machine

Key Impairments Addressed:
1. Decreased proximal strength
2. Decreased distal strength
3. Decreased pinch grip
4. Decreased fine motor control

Materials:
Coins
Coin bank placed on its side to simulate orientation of vending machine coin slot

Task Description:
1. Grasp coin and pick up from table with affected hand.
2. Place in slot of coin bank.

Grading Task:

Increase difficulty	Decrease difficulty
Use small coins, such as dimes or pennies. • Requires more fine motor control.	Use large coins. • Requires less fine motor control.
Select bank with small coin slot. • Requires more fine motor control.	Select bank with large coin slot or have client place coin into cup. • Requires less fine motor control.
Stand, with bank on overhead shelf. • Requires more proximal strength and motor control.	Sit, with bank placed on table. • Requires less proximal strength and motor control.

Task Mastery:
1. Consistently grasps coin and places into slot on first attempt.
2. Does not drop coin.

Ideas for related tasks	Rationale
Writing on chalkboard or dry-erase board	Requires proximal and distal strength. Requires proximal and fine motor control.
Stacking books vertically on shelf	Requires proximal and distal strength. Requires proximal motor control.
Pinning thumbtack to bulletin board	Requires distal strength and pinch grip. Requires proximal and fine motor control.

50. Task: Retrieving wallet from pocket

Key Impairments Addressed:
1. Decreased proximal strength
2. Decreased grip strength
3. Decreased distal motor control

Materials:
Wallet
Pants pocket

Task Description:
1. Stand with wallet in pocket.
2. Reach into pocket with affected hand to retrieve wallet.
3. Set on table, then grasp again and replace in pocket.

Grading Task:

Increase difficulty	Decrease difficulty
Wear pants with narrow, deep pocket.	Wear pants with wide, shallow pocket.
• Requires more grip strength.	• Requires less grip strength.
• Requires more distal motor control.	• Requires less distal motor control.
Retrieve wallet from back pocket.	Retrieve wallet from side pocket.
• Requires more proximal strength.	• Requires less proximal strength.

Task Mastery:
1. Reaches into pocket and grasps wallet on first attempt.
2. Places wallet into pocket without dropping.

Ideas for related tasks	Rationale
Threading belt through belt loops	Requires grip strength. Requires distal motor control.
Tucking shirt into back of pants	Requires proximal strength. Requires distal strength and motor control.

51. Task: Retrieving bills from billfold

Key Impairments Addressed:
1. Decreased pinch grip
2. Decreased distal motor control

Materials:
Billfold or wallet
Dollar bills

Task Description:
1. Hold billfold in unaffected hand.
2. Grasp bill with affected hand and set on table.
3. Place bill back into billfold with affected hand.

Grading Task:

Increase difficulty	Decrease difficulty
Retrieve folded bills from wallet.	Retrieve group of bills from wallet.
• Requires more distal motor control.	• Requires less distal motor control.
Retrieve one bill from among many bills in wallet.	Retrieve one bill from otherwise empty wallet.
• Requires more distal motor control.	• Requires less distal motor control.

Task Mastery:
1. Consistently grasps bill in billfold on first attempt.

Ideas for related tasks	Rationale
Organizing receipts	Requires pinch grip. Requires distal motor control.
Sorting pills	Requires pinch grip. Requires fine motor control.

52. Task: Dialing telephone number

Key Impairments Addressed:
1. Decreased distal strength
2. Decreased fine motor control

Materials:
Telephone

Task Description:
1. Grasp telephone with unaffected hand, and dial telephone numbers with affected hand.
2. After dialing a telephone number, set the phone down.

Grading Task:

Increase difficulty	Decrease difficulty
Pick telephone up with affected hand, and dial number with thumb of affected hand. • Requires more distal strength and fine motor control.	Pick telephone up and set down with unaffected hand. • Requires less distal strength and fine motor control.
Use a telephone with small buttons, such as a cell phone. • Requires more fine motor control.	Use a telephone with large buttons, such as an office phone. • Requires less fine motor control.

Task Mastery:
1. Consistently selects correct number on dial pad on first attempt.

Ideas for related tasks	Rationale
Sending a text message	Requires distal strength. Requires fine motor control.
Using a remote control	Requires distal strength. Requires fine motor control.

53. Task: Turning steering wheel

Key Impairments Addressed:
1. Decreased proximal strength
2. Decreased grip strength
3. Decreased distal motor control

Materials:
Steering wheel

Task Description:
1. Grasp steering wheel.
2. Turn to right and left; release.

Grading Task:

Increase difficulty	Decrease difficulty
Increase arc of turn in both directions. • Requires more distal motor control.	Decrease arc of turn in both directions. • Requires less distal motor control.
Change hand position on steering wheel. • Requires more proximal strength and motor control.	Place hands in desired spot on steering wheel. • Requires less proximal strength and motor control.

Task Mastery:
1. Consistently grasps and releases wheel on first attempt

Ideas for related tasks	Rationale
Rolling dice	Requires distal strength and motor control.
Shaking small bottle of juice	Requires grip strength. Requires distal motor control.

54. Task: Turning oven dial or timer

Key Impairments Addressed:
1. Decreased distal strength
2. Decreased pinch grip
3. Decreased distal motor control

Materials:
Dial or timer

Task Description:
1. Reach for dial with affected arm, and turn to set time or temperature.
2. Release grip; return arm to side and repeat.

Grading Task:

Increase difficulty	Decrease difficulty
Use small dial placed arm's length away from client.	Use timer placed on table in front of client.
• Requires more proximal strength and motor control.	• Requires less proximal strength and motor control.
Use tight dial that is more difficult to turn.	Use loose or easily turned dial.
• Requires more distal strength and pinch grip.	• Requires less distal strength and pinch grip.

Task Mastery:
1. Consistently grasps and turns dial to desired setting on first attempt.

Ideas for related tasks	Rationale
Turning radio dial	Requires pinch grip.
	Requires distal motor control.
Setting timer	Requires pinch grip.
	Requires distal motor control.
Locking door	Requires pinch grip.
	Requires distal motor control.

55. Task: Fastening clothes to clothesline

Key Impairments Addressed:
1. Decreased proximal strength
2. Decreased pinch grip
3. Decreased proximal motor control
4. Decreased fine motor control

Materials:
Clothes
Clothespin
Clothesline

Task Description:
1. Grasp clothespin with affected hand and article of clothing with unaffected hand.
2. Fasten article to clothesline with clothespin.

Grading Task:

Increase difficulty	Decrease difficulty
Use small or stiff clothespin. • Requires more pinch grip. • Requires more fine motor control.	Use large, adapted clothespin. • Requires less pinch grip. • Requires less fine motor control.
Raise the height of the clothesline. • Requires more proximal strength and motor control.	Lower the height of the clothesline. • Requires less proximal strength and motor control.
	Grasp clothing with affected hand and pin with unaffected hand. • Requires no pinch grip.

Task Mastery:
1. Consistently pinches clothespin to fasten clothes on first attempt without dropping.

Ideas for related tasks	Rationale
Fastening binder clip to papers	Require pinch grip. Requires fine motor control.
Hanging clothes on hanger	Requires proximal strength and grip strength. Requires proximal motor control.

56. Task: Opening containers

Key Impairments Addressed:
1. Decreased distal strength
2. Decreased grip strength

Materials:
Containers

Note. Many types of containers can be used, such as plastic storage containers, spice bottles, soda bottles, butter tubs, and so forth.

Task Description:
1. Grasp lid with affected hand and container with unaffected hand.
2. Place lid on container using affected hand, then remove.

Note. This is an example of a task in which the affected hand could be trained as the stabilizing or opening hand, depending on the eventual goal.

Grading Task:

Increase difficulty	Decrease difficulty
Vary the size of and type of container. • Requires more distal strength.	Use containers requiring the same type of grip. • Requires less distal strength.
Fill containers to top. • Requires more distal motor control.	Open empty container. • Requires less distal motor control.
Retrieve containers from shelf with affected upper extremity before opening • Requires proximal strength.	Set containers on front of table. • Requires less proximal strength.

Task Mastery:
1. Consistently grasps lid and places on and removes from plastic storage container on first attempt.

Ideas for related tasks	Rationale
Opening toothpaste tube	Requires distal strength and grip strength.
Removing lid from jug	Requires distal strength and grip strength.

57. Task: Pouring cereal from box

Key Impairments Addressed:
1. Decreased proximal strength
2. Decreased grip strength
3. Decreased proximal motor control
4. Decreased distal motor control

Materials:
Cereal box
Bowl

Task Description:
1. Grasp cereal box and remove from shelf of cabinet using affected arm.
2. Pour small amount of cereal into a bowl, then replace box on shelf and repeat.

Grading Task:

Increase difficulty	Decrease difficulty
Increase height of shelf on which box is placed. • Requires more proximal strength.	Set box on table in front of client. • Requires less proximal strength.
Pour cereal into small, narrow bowl. • Requires more distal motor control.	Pour cereal into large bowl. • Requires less distal motor control.
Use large, wide cereal box. • Requires more distal strength.	Use individual-sized cereal box. • Requires less distal strength.

Task Mastery:
1. Consistently grasps box and pours cereal into bowl without spilling.
2. Does not drop box.

Idea for related task	Rationale
Pouring juice from carton	Requires proximal strength and grip strength. Requires proximal and distal motor control.

58. Task: Opening resealable plastic bag

Key Impairments Addressed:
1. Decreased pinch grip
2. Decreased fine motor control

Materials:
Resealable plastic bags

Task Description:
1. Grasp two sides of bag and pull apart.
2. Set bag down, then grasp again and repeat.

Grading Task:

Increase difficulty	Decrease difficulty
Use a small bag.	Use a large bag.
• Requires more fine motor control.	• Requires less fine motor control.
Pull bag out of box in which it is stored.	Set individual bag on table.
• Requires more fine motor control.	• Requires less fine motor control.

Task Mastery:
1. Consistently grasps bag and opens on first attempt.

Ideas for related tasks	Rationale
Zipping jacket	Requires pinch grip and fine motor control.
Sealing an envelope	Requires pinch grip and fine motor control.
Opening a bandage	Requires pinch grip and fine motor control.

59. Task: Tying grocery bag

Key Impairments Addressed:
1. Decreased distal strength
2. Decreased grip strength
3. Decreased fine motor control

Materials:
Grocery sacks

Task Description:
1. Stand with grocery bag containing items on countertop.
2. Tie bag with bilateral hands.
3. Untie bag.

Grading Task:

Increase difficulty	Decrease difficulty
Hold bag in the air to tie. • Requires more proximal strength.	Sit down with bag on lap. • Requires less proximal strength.
Fill bag to top, then tie. • Requires more fine motor control.	Tie bag with few items inside. • Requires less fine motor control.
Double knot the bag. • Requires more fine motor control.	Single knot the bag. • Requires less fine motor control.

Task Mastery:
1. Consistently grasps bag and ties into knot on first attempt.

Ideas for related tasks	Rationale
Fastening a bag with a twist tie	Requires grip strength. Requires fine motor control.
Tying shoes	Requires grip strength. Requires fine motor control.

60. Task: Packing and unpacking backpack

Key Impairments Addressed:
1. Decreased proximal strength
2. Decreased distal strength
3. Decreased grip strength
4. Decreased distal motor control

Materials:
Backpack
Books or other items packed into bag

Task Description:
1. Hold backpack open with unaffected hand.
2. Grasp items one by one with affected hand and place into backpack.
3. Zip with affected hand.
4. Unzip and remove items with affected hand; repeat.

Grading Task:

Increase difficulty	Decrease difficulty
Use backpack with many small pockets in which items can be placed. • Requires more distal strength and motor control.	Use backpack with one large pocket. • Requires less distal strength and motor control.
Select heavy items to place into backpack (e.g., books, full water bottle). • Requires more proximal strength and grip strength.	Select lightweight items to place into backpack. • Requires less proximal strength and grip strength.

Task Mastery:
1. Grasps items with affected hand and places in backpack without dropping.
2. Zips backpack with affected hand on first attempt.

Idea for related task	Rationale
Filling grocery bags	Requires proximal and distal strength. Requires distal motor control.

61. Task: Tacking paper to bulletin board

Key Impairments Addressed:
1. Decreased proximal strength
2. Decreased pinch grip
3. Decreased distal motor control

Materials:
Thumbtacks
Bulletin board

Task Description:
1. Grasp paper with unaffected hand and thumbtack with affected hand.
2. Tack paper to board; repeat.

Grading Task:

Increase difficulty	Decrease difficulty
Use small thumbtacks.	Use large thumbtacks.
• Requires more pinch grip.	• Requires less pinch grip.
• Requires more distal motor control.	• Requires less distal motor control.
Tack paper overhead and in various spots off to the side of the board.	Tack paper on board in front at shoulder height.
• Requires more proximal strength and motor control.	• Requires less proximal strength and motor control.

Task Mastery:
1. Consistently grasps thumbtack on first attempt and inserts into board.
2. Does not drop thumbtack.

Idea for related task	Rationale
Fastening paper on refrigerator with a magnet	Requires proximal strength and motor control. Requires pinch grip.

62. Task: Dusting table

Key Impairments Addressed:
1. Decreased proximal strength
2. Decreased grip strength
3. Decreased distal motor control

Materials:
Dust rag
Table

Task Description:
1. Grasp dust rag with affected hand.
2. Wipe table, making three to four strokes, then pull rag off of table and repeat.

Grading Task:

Increase difficulty	Decrease difficulty
Make large, circular motions with rag on table. • Requires more proximal strength and motor control.	Dust back and forth, making small motions. • Requires less proximal strength and motor control.
Dust tall bookshelf. • Requires more proximal strength.	

Task Mastery:
1. Consistently grasps dust rag and wipes table with smooth motion.

Ideas for related tasks	Rationale
Wiping windows	Requires proximal strength and motor control.
Cleaning table	Requires proximal strength and motor control.
Sanding wall	Requires proximal strength and grip strength. Requires proximal motor control.

63. Task: Stacking laundry

Key Impairments Addressed:
1. Decreased proximal strength
2. Decreased distal strength
3. Decreased distal motor control

Materials:
Clothes
Laundry basket

Task Description:
1. Grasp stack of towels with affected hand below stack and unaffected hand above.
2. Lift towels out of laundry basket and onto table top.
3. Repeat, setting stack back into basket.

Grading Task:

Increase difficulty	Decrease difficulty
Increase the size of the stack. • Requires more proximal strength and motor control for added weight.	Decrease the size of the stack. • Requires less proximal strength and motor control.
Lift stack from basket placed on chair and walk it to countertop. • Requires more proximal and distal strength.	Move stack from one spot on table to another. • Requires less proximal and distal strength.

Task Mastery:
1. Consistently grasps stack of laundry with effective hand placement and lifts onto table or places in laundry basket without dropping.

Ideas for related tasks	Rationale
Moving boxes	Requires proximal and distal strength.
Stacking plates in cabinet	Requires proximal and distal strength. Requires proximal and distal motor control.

64. Task: Stacking books on bookshelf

Key Impairments Addressed:
1. Decreased proximal strength
2. Decreased grip strength
3. Decreased proximal motor control

Materials:
Books
Bookshelf

Task Description:
1. Grasp book with affected hand.
2. Place onto bookshelf and repeat.

Grading Task:

Increase difficulty	Decrease difficulty
Alternate between stacking books upright and flat. • Requires more distal strength and motor control.	Stack books flat on shelf. • Requires less distal strength and motor control.
Stack books on elevated shelf. • Requires more proximal strength and motor control.	Stack books on low shelf. • Requires less proximal strength and motor control.
Stack heavy textbooks. • Requires more proximal strength and grip strength.	Stack lightweight paperback books. • Requires less proximal strength and grip strength.

Task Mastery:
1. Consistently grasps book with effective grip and places on bookshelf without dropping.
2. Places book in desired spot on each attempt.

Ideas for related tasks	Rationale
Stacking plates in cabinet	Requires proximal strength and grip strength. Requires proximal motor control.
Placing groceries in cabinet	Requires proximal strength and grip strength. Requires proximal motor control.

65. Task: Chopping vegetables

Key Impairments Addressed:
1. Decreased grip strength
2. Decreased distal motor control

Materials:
Vegetables, putty, or similar item to cut
Knife
Cutting board

Task Description:
1. Grasp knife with affected hand and fork with unaffected hand (or no fork, depending on the item being cut).
2. Stabilize food with fork (if necessary) while cutting with knife.
3. Set silverware down and repeat.

Grading Task:

Increase difficulty	Decrease difficulty
Use standard-sized paring knife. • Requires more grip strength.	Use adaptive knife, such as rocker knife. • Requires less grip strength and distal motor control.
Select items that are firm, such as carrot, celery, or stiff putty. • Requires more grip strength and distal strength.	Select softer items, such as play dough or bread. • Requires less grip strength and distal strength.

Task Mastery:
1. Grasps knife with effective grasp on first attempt.
2. Cuts.

Idea for related task	Rationale
Slicing pizza	Requires grip strength. Requires proximal motor control.

66. Task: Emptying trash can

Key Impairments Addressed:
1. Decreased proximal strength
2. Decreased distal strength

Materials:
Small trash can
Large trash can or other target

Task Description:
1. Grasp small trash can with bilateral hands.
2. Tip upside down over large trash can to empty.
3. Return to floor and repeat.

Grading Task:

Increase difficulty	Decrease difficulty
Use large trash can. • Requires more proximal strength.	Use small trash can. • Requires less proximal strength.
Use full trash can. • Requires more proximal strength and motor control to keep can steady while lifting.	Use empty trash can. • Requires less proximal strength and motor control.
Use tall trash can. • Requires more proximal strength and motor control to lift small can over edge of large can.	Use short trash can. • Requires less proximal strength and motor control.

Task Mastery:
1. Consistently grasps and tips trash can over on first attempt without dropping.
2. Does not drop can.

Ideas for related tasks	Rationale
Lifting box	Requires proximal and distal strength.
Lifting laundry basket	Requires proximal and distal strength.

67. Task: Placing trash bag into trash can

Key Impairments Addressed:
1. Decreased proximal strength
2. Decreased grip strength
3. Decreased proximal motor control

Materials:
Trash bag
Trash can

Task Description:
1. Grasp trash bag and lift from container.
2. Open it and place it into trash can with bilateral hands.

Grading Task:

Increase difficulty	Decrease difficulty
Use large trash bag and trash can. • Requires more proximal motor control.	Use small trash bag and trash can. • Requires less proximal motor control.
Retrieve trash bag from elevated or under-counter shelf. • Requires more proximal strength.	Retrieve trash bag from tabletop. • Requires less proximal strength.

Task Mastery:
1. Consistently grasps bag and places into can on first attempt.
2. Does not drop bag.

Ideas for related tasks	Rationale
Laying blanket out on ground	Requires proximal strength and grip strength. Requires proximal motor control.
Shaking out towel	Requires proximal strength and grip strength. Requires proximal motor control.

68. Task: Grasping paper towel from roll

Key Impairments Addressed:
1. Decreased proximal strength
2. Decreased grip strength

Materials:
Paper towels
Paper towel holder

Task Description:
1. Stand at countertop and pull paper towel off of roll.

Grading Task:

Increase difficulty	Decrease difficulty
Place dispenser on shelf or attach underneath cabinet.	Place dispenser on edge of table.
• Requires more proximal strength.	• Requires less proximal strength.
Pull off several sheets at a time.	Pull off one sheet at a time.
• Requires more proximal strength to pull towels out.	• Requires less proximal strength to pull towels out.

Task Mastery:
1. Consistently grasps towel on first attempt.
2. Demonstrates smooth trajectory of movement during reach toward paper towels.

Ideas for related tasks	Rationale
Grasping foil and pulling from roll	Requires proximal strength and grip strength.
Grasping garbage bag and pulling from roll	Requires proximal strength and grip strength.
Grasping plastic wrap and pulling from roll	Requires proximal strength and grip strength.

69. Task: Donning headphones

Key Impairments Addressed:
1. Decreased proximal strength
2. Decreased grip strength

Materials:
Headphones

Task Description:
1. Grasp headphones and place on ears.

Grading Task:

Increase difficulty	Decrease difficulty
Use small earbuds.	Use large headphones.
• Requires more fine motor control.	• Requires less fine motor control.

Task Mastery:
1. Consistently grasps and places headphones on ears on first attempt.

Ideas for related tasks	Rationale
Donning earmuffs	Requires proximal strength and grip strength.
Donning earrings	Requires proximal strength and grip strength. Requires fine motor control.

70. Task: Spreading peanut butter onto bread

Key Impairments Addressed:
1. Decreased grip strength
2. Decreased distal motor control

Materials:
Bread (or nonfood item of similar size and weight as bread)
Knife
Peanut butter
Plate

Task Description:
1. Hold slice of bread with unaffected hand.
2. Use affected hand to grasp knife and lift from plate.
3. Dip into condiment jar and spread onto bread.
4. Set knife down on plate and repeat.

Note. May use squeeze bottle requiring tipping upside down (i.e., ketchup bottle) to address other impairments such as decreased gross grip strength, wrist strength, or forearm pronation.

Grading Task:

Increase difficulty	Decrease difficulty
Use nearly empty peanut butter jar. • Requires more distal strength and motor control.	Use full peanut butter jar. • Requires less distal strength and motor control.
Use small knife. • Requires more grip strength and distal motor control.	Use large knife or spoon. • Requires less grip strength and distal motor control.
Stabilize jar on table for scooping. • Requires more distal strength and motor control.	Lift jar off of table and tilt for easier access into jar with affected hand. • Requires less distal strength and motor control.

Task Mastery:
1. Consistently scoops sufficient amount of peanut butter onto knife and spreads.
2. Consistently grasps knife on first attempt.

Ideas for related tasks	Rationale
Squeezing or shaking condiment out of bottle (i.e., ketchup bottle)	Requires grip strength and distal motor control.
Squeezing toothpaste out of tube	Requires grip strength and distal motor control.
Dipping paintbrush into paint can	Requires grip strength and distal motor control.

71. Task: Using calculator

Key Impairments Addressed:
1. Decreased distal strength
2. Decreased distal motor control

Materials:
Calculator

Task Description:
1. Open calculator with bilateral hands.
2. Type numbers into calculator.

Grading Task:

Increase difficulty	Decrease difficulty
Use small pocket calculator.	Use large calculator.
• Requires more distal motor control.	• Requires less distal motor control.
Type long numbers or equations.	Type numbers with few digits.
• Requires more distal motor control.	• Requires less distal motor control.

Task Mastery:
1. Consistently presses correct numbers on each attempt.

Ideas for related tasks	Rationale
Typing a text message	Requires distal strength and motor control.
Dialing a phone	Requires distal strength and motor control.

72. Task: Wrapping food in foil

Key Impairments Addressed:
1. Decreased distal strength
2. Decreased grip strength

Materials:
Foil
Items simulating food

Task Description:
1. Pull foil off of roll.
2. Set simulated food item on foil and wrap.

Grading Task:

Increase difficulty	Decrease difficulty
Use large piece of foil.	Use small piece of foil.
• Requires more proximal strength.	• Requires less proximal strength.

Task Mastery:
1. Consistently pulls foil off of roll on first attempt.
2. Grasps foil for wrapping on first attempt.

Ideas for related tasks	Rationale
Wrapping a present	Requires distal strength and grip strength. Requires distal motor control.
Making a bed	Requires proximal and distal strength.
Tearing plastic wrap off of roll	Requires distal strength and grip strength.

73. Task: Setting microwave

Key Impairments Addressed:
1. Decreased proximal strength
2. Decreased proximal motor control
3. Decreased distal motor control

Materials:
Microwave

Task Description:
1. Set microwave to desired time.

Grading Task:

Increase difficulty	Decrease difficulty
Place microwave on shelf or above stove.	Place microwave on table.
• Requires more proximal strength.	• Requires less proximal strength.

Task Mastery:
1. Consistently presses correct buttons on first attempt.

Ideas for related tasks	Rationale
Using calculator	Requires distal motor control.
Sending a text message	Requires distal motor control.
Pressing numbers on ATM or vending machine	Requires distal motor control.

74. Task: Squeezing dish soap from bottle

Key Impairments Addressed:
1. Decreased distal strength
2. Decreased grip strength
3. Decreased distal motor control

Materials:
Bottle of dish soap

Task Description:
1. Grasp dish soap bottle.
2. Tip and squeeze into sink.
3. Replace on sink and repeat.

Grading Task:

Increase difficulty	Decrease difficulty
Use wide soap bottle. • Requires more distal strength.	Use small, narrow soap bottle. • Requires less distal strength.
Note. Could decrease difficulty if grip strength is more impaired than finger extension.	*Note.* Could increase difficulty if grip strength is more impaired than finger extension.
Use heavy soap bottle. • Requires more distal strength and grip strength.	Use lightweight bottle. • Requires less distal strength and grip strength.
Use bottle that is nearly empty. • Requires more distal motor control.	Use bottle that is full. • Requires less distal motor control.

Task Mastery:
1. Consistently grasps and releases bottle on first attempt.
2. Consistently tips bottle upside down and squeezes soap out without dropping.

Ideas for related tasks	Rationale
Squeezing syrup onto plate	Requires distal strength and grip strength.
Squeezing ketchup onto hamburger bun	Requires distal strength and grip strength.

75. Task: Pouring detergent into dishwasher

Key Impairments Addressed:
1. Decreased distal strength
2. Decreased grip strength
3. Decreased distal motor control

Materials:
Detergent
Cup placed below knee level to simulate dishwasher detergent cup

Task Description:
1. Grasp dishwashing detergent box or bottle with affected hand.
2. Pour into dishwasher cup or in small cup placed below waist level.

Grading Task:

Increase difficulty	Decrease difficulty
Use wide box of detergent. • Requires more distal strength.	Use small, narrow box. • Requires less distal strength.
Use heavy box or bottle. • Requires more grip strength.	Use lightweight box or bottle. • Requires less grip strength.

Task Mastery:
1. Consistently pours detergent into cup without spilling.
2. Grasps and releases detergent box or bottle on first attempt.

Ideas for related tasks	Rationale
Pouring food into dog bowl	Requires distal strength and grip strength. Requires distal motor control.
Pouring dirt into flower pot	Requires distal strength and grip strength. Requires distal motor control.

76. Task: Pouring detergent into washing machine

Key Impairments Addressed:
1. Decreased proximal strength
2. Decreased grip strength
3. Decreased distal motor control

Materials:
Laundry detergent
Sink or bucket

Task Description:
1. Grasp laundry detergent with unaffected hand.
2. Untwist and hold measuring cup with affected hand, and pour detergent into cup.
3. Pour detergent from lid into washing machine (use sink or bucket to simulate machine) using affected hand.

Grading Task:

Increase difficulty	Decrease difficulty
Pour large amount of detergent into cup for added weight. • Requires more grip strength.	Do not pour detergent into cup. • Requires less grip strength.
Secure cap firmly on detergent. • Requires more distal strength and grip strength to untwist cap.	Place cap loosely on detergent. • Requires less distal strength and grip strength.
Use deep cup. • Requires more distal strength during pouring.	Use shallow cup or cup with pouring spout. • Requires less distal strength.

Task Mastery:
1. Consistently removes measuring cup without dropping.
2. Stabilizes cup and pours detergent into machine without dropping.

Ideas for related tasks	Rationale
Pouring measuring cup of flour into mixing bowl	Requires distal strength and grip strength. Requires distal motor control.

77. Task: Adjusting rearview mirror in car

Key Impairments Addressed:
1. Decreased proximal strength
2. Decreased grip strength
3. Decreased distal motor control

Materials:
Rearview mirror of car or simulated position of mirror

Task Description:
1. Reach up to rearview mirror in car with affected hand, move three to four times, and return arm to lap.

Grading Task:

Increase difficulty	Decrease difficulty
Tighten mirror so it is stiffer to adjust. • Requires more grip strength.	Loosen mirror so it is less stiff to adjust. • Requires less grip strength.
Move mirror widely to sides. • Requires more distal motor control.	Move mirror through small motions. • Requires less distal motor control.

Task Mastery:
1. Consistently grasps mirror on first attempt.
2. Moves to desired position and releases hand on first attempt.

Idea for related task	Rationale
Adjusting cosmetic mirror on table	Requires proximal strength and grip strength.

78. Task: Slicing pizza

Key Impairments Addressed:
1. Decreased proximal strength
2. Decreased grip strength
3. Decreased proximal motor control

Materials:
Pizza slicer
Cutting board
Putty to cut

Task Description:
1. Grasp pizza slicer with affected hand.
2. Roll slicer back and forth through pizza or putty three to four times.
3. Set slicer down and repeat.

Grading Task:

Increase difficulty	Decrease difficulty
Use thick putty to slice. • Requires more proximal strength and grip strength.	Use thin putty or play dough that is less stiff. • Requires less proximal strength and grip strength.
Use pizza slicer with thin handle. • Requires more grip strength.	Use pizza slicer with adaptive handle. • Requires less grip strength.

Task Mastery:
1. Grasps and releases slicer on first attempt.
2. Makes cuts with slicer on each attempt.

Ideas for related tasks	Rationale
Slicing bread	Requires proximal strength and motor control. Requires grip strength.
Chopping vegetables	Requires grip strength. Requires distal motor control.

79. Task: Peeling vegetables

Key Impairments Addressed:
1. Decreased distal strength
2. Decreased grip strength
3. Decreased distal motor control

Materials:
Vegetables
Vegetable peeler

Task Description:
1. Grasp vegetable with unaffected hand and peeler with affected hand.
2. Peel vegetable three to four times, then set peeler down and repeat.

Note. This is an example of a task in which the affected hand could be trained as the grasping hand, not the peeling hand, depending on the eventual goal.

Grading Task:

Increase difficulty	Decrease difficulty
Use thin-handled peeler. • Requires more grip strength.	Use peeler with adapted handle. • Requires less grip strength.
Stand and hold vegetable over table, over sink, or in the air to peel. • Requires more grip strength. • Requires more distal motor control.	Sit at table and stabilize arms on tabletop while peeling. • Requires less grip strength. • Requires less distal motor control.

Task Mastery:
1. Effectively peels vegetable with each stroke.
2. Does not drop peeler.

Ideas for related tasks	Rationale
Scrubbing dishes with dish-washing wand	Requires distal strength and grip strength. Requires distal motor control.
Sharpening knife with knife sharpener	Requires distal strength and grip strength. Requires distal motor control.

80. Task: Placing cookie sheet into oven

Key Impairments Addressed:
1. Decreased proximal strength
2. Decreased distal strength

Materials:
Cookie sheet
Oven or shelf positioned below waist level

Task Description:
1. Grasp cookie sheet with affected hand.
2. Place on shelf in oven.
3. Don oven mitt, and remove sheet from oven.
4. Doff oven mitt, and repeat steps.

Note. Keep oven turned off for safety.

Grading Task:

Increase difficulty	Decrease difficulty
Use heavy cookie sheet. • Requires more distal strength.	Use small or lightweight cookie sheet. • Requires less distal strength.
Place on bottom shelf of oven. • Requires more distal motor control.	Place on top shelf of oven. • Requires less distal motor control.
Place items on cookie sheet that may slide around if sheet is not held flat. • Requires more distal strength and motor control.	Do not set anything on cookie sheet. • Requires less distal strength and motor control.

Task Mastery:
1. Consistently grasps and releases cookie sheet on first attempt.
2. Consistently dons and doffs oven mitt on first attempt.

Ideas for related tasks	Rationale
Unloading dishwasher	Requires proximal and distal strength. Requires grip strength with arm positioned below waist level.
Placing pots and pans in low cabinet or drawer below oven	Requires proximal and distal strength. Requires grip strength with arm positioned below waist level.

81. Task: Mailing a letter

Key Impairments Addressed:
1. Decreased distal strength
2. Decreased grip strength

Materials:
Paper
Envelope
Stamp or sticker

Task Description:
1. Use bilateral hands to fold a letter into thirds.
2. Use affected hand to insert letter into envelope.
3. Use affected hand to place stamp (or sticker or sticky note) on letter.
4. Seal envelope and place in mailbox or other small box using affected arm.

Grading Task:

Increase difficulty	Decrease difficulty
Fold letter into fourths and use small envelope. • Requires more distal strength.	Use large 8½" × 11" envelope, and do not fold letter. • Requires less distal strength.
Use thick, heavy paper, such as cardstock. • Requires more distal strength.	Use standard-weight paper. • Requires less distal strength.
Place in mailbox at shoulder height. • Requires more proximal strength.	Place in mailbox at table height. • Requires less proximal strength.

Task Mastery:
1. Consistently folds paper and places in envelope on first attempt.
2. Places in mailbox without dropping.

Idea for related task	Rationale
Folding a handkerchief	Requires distal strength. Requires grip strength.

82. Task: Fastening twist tie to bread bag

Key Impairments Addressed:
1. Decreased pinch grip
2. Decreased fine motor control

Materials:
Twist tie
Bag

Task Description:
1. Grasp tie with affected hand and twist around bag.
2. Use affected hand to untwist the tie, and set it back down on table.

Grading Task:

Increase difficulty	Decrease difficulty
Use small, stiff twist tie.	Use large, loose twist tie.
• Requires more pinch grip.	• Requires less pinch grip.
• Requires more fine motor control.	• Requires less fine motor control.
Stand, holding bag in air while twisting tie.	Sit at table or rest bag on counter to fasten tie to bag.
• Requires more proximal strength.	• Requires less proximal strength.
• Requires more distal motor control.	• Requires less distal motor control.

Task Mastery:
1. Grasps, releases, and ties on first attempt.
2. Does not drop twist tie.

Idea for related task	Rationale
Fastening chip clip to bag	Requires grip strength.

83. Task: Using rolling pin

Key Impairments Addressed:
1. Decreased proximal strength
2. Decreased grip strength

Materials:
Rolling pin
Putty or other material to roll

Task Description:
1. Grasp rolling pin, and roll back and forth.

Grading Task:

Increase difficulty	Decrease difficulty
Use rolling pin with small handles. • Requires more grip strength.	Use rolling pin with built-up handles. • Requires less grip strength.
Use stiff putty or material that is difficult to press. • Requires more proximal strength and grip strength.	Use soft, pliable material. • Requires less proximal strength and grip strength.

Task Mastery:
1. Consistently grasps and releases handles on first attempt.
2. Demonstrates smooth, coordinated motion during rolling.

Idea for related task	Rationale
Kneading dough	Requires grip strength.

84. Task: Raking leaves

Key Impairments Addressed:
1. Decreased proximal strength
2. Decreased grip strength

Materials:
Rake
Leaves

Task Description:
1. Grasp rake and rake leaves (or scraps of paper to simulate leaves) into piles.

Grading Task:

Increase difficulty	Decrease difficulty
Use large, heavy rake.	Use small, lightweight rake.
• Requires more proximal strength and grip strength.	• Requires less proximal strength and grip strength.
Bag leaves or paper after raking.	
• Requires more proximal strength and grip strength.	

Task Mastery:
1. Consistently grasps and releases rake on first attempt.
2. Demonstrates coordinated movement during raking.

Ideas for related tasks	Rationale
Sweeping floor	Requires proximal strength and grip strength.
Shoveling snow	Requires proximal and distal strength. Requires grip strength.

85. Task: Watering plants

Key Impairments Addressed:
1. Decreased proximal strength
2. Decreased grip strength

Materials:
Watering can
Plants

Task Description:
1. Grasp watering can and pour water onto plants.

Grading Task:

Increase difficulty	Decrease difficulty
Fill watering can to the top with water. • Requires more proximal strength and grip strength. • Requires more proximal and distal motor control.	Simulate pouring with empty watering can. • Requires less proximal strength and grip strength. • Requires less proximal and distal motor control.
Water plants in hanging baskets. • Requires more proximal strength and motor control.	Water plants on tabletop. • Requires less proximal strength and motor control.

Task Mastery:
1. Consistently grasps and releases can on first attempt.
2. Does not drop can.

Ideas for related tasks	Rationale
Pouring juice from pitcher	Requires proximal strength and grip strength. Requires proximal and distal motor control.
Pouring cereal	Requires proximal strength and grip strength. Requires proximal and distal motor control.

Exhibit 4.5. Leisure Tasks

86. Task: Casting fishing line

Key Impairments Addressed:
1. Decreased proximal strength
2. Decreased grip strength
3. Decreased proximal and distal motor control

Materials:
Fishing pole

Task Description:
1. Stand and grasp fishing pole with affected hand.
2. Simulate casting by flipping pole forward.
3. Turn reel with unaffected hand to bring in fishing line (if safe in setting).

Note. This is an example of a task in which the affected hand could be trained as the reeling hand rather than the grasping hand, depending on the eventual goal.

Grading Task:

Increase difficulty	Decrease difficulty
Use longer fishing line.	Use short fishing line.
• Requires more proximal strength to cast line.	• Requires less proximal strength to cast line.
Use heavy fishing pole.	Use lightweight fishing pole.
• Requires more proximal and grip strength.	• Requires less proximal and grip strength.

Task Mastery:
1. Consistently grasps pole and casts line on first attempt.
2. Demonstrates smooth trajectory of movement during casting.

Ideas for related tasks	Rationale
Swinging tennis racquet	Requires proximal and distal strength.
	Requires proximal and distal motor control.
Swinging baseball bat	Requires proximal and distal strength.
	Requires proximal and distal motor control.

87. Task: Scrapbooking

Key Impairments Addressed:
1. Decreased distal strength
2. Decreased grip strength
3. Decreased fine motor control

Materials:
Book
Paper
Photos
Scissors
Glue

Task Description:
1. Hold items with affected hand while using scissors or glue with unaffected hand.
2. Place items into scrapbook with affected hand.

Note. Take necessary safety precautions if requiring client to use scissors and glue. Consider using scissors in opposite hand, using children's scissors and glue, or both.

Grading Task:

Increase difficulty	Decrease difficulty
Use small materials, such as stickers. • Requires more fine motor control.	Use large materials, such as thick paper. • Requires less fine motor control.
Use decorative scissors in affected hand to cut scrapbook paper and photos. • Requires more fine motor control.	Avoid using scissors by using paper and photos as they are or use scissors in unaffected hand. • Requires less fine motor control.
Use affected extremity to reach for and grasp items. • Requires more distal strength.	Use unaffected extremity to reach for and grasp items; stabilize items with affected hand. • Requires less distal strength.

Task Mastery:
1. Consistently cuts and pastes items in proper spot on first attempt.
2. Does not drop items.

Ideas for related tasks	Rationale
Filling a photo album	Requires distal strength. Requires fine motor control.
Doing arts and crafts	Requires distal strength. Requires fine motor control.

88. Task: Rolling dice

Key Impairments Addressed:
1. Decreased distal strength
2. Decreased fine motor control

Materials:
Dice

Task Description:
1. Grasp dice on table.
2. Shake in palm.
3. Roll onto table.

Grading Task:

Increase difficulty	Decrease difficulty
Increase number of dice grasped and rolled. • Requires more fine motor control.	Use only one die. • Requires less fine motor control.
Roll dice onto small target, such as small board game. • Requires more distal motor control.	Roll dice onto large tabletop. • Requires less distal motor control.

Task Mastery:
1. Consistently grasps and then releases dice on first attempt.
2. Consistently hits target when rolling dice.

Idea for related task	Rationale
Emptying change from pockets or purse	Requires distal strength and motor control.

89. Task: Playing cards

Key Impairments Addressed:
1. Decreased proximal strength
2. Decreased pinch grip
3. Decreased proximal motor control
4. Decreased distal motor control

Materials:
Deck of playing cards

Task Description:
1. Hold deck in unaffected hand.
2. Grasp card with affected hand and place on table or hand to practitioner.

Grading Task:

Increase difficulty	Decrease difficulty
Use smaller deck of cards. • Requires more fine motor control.	Use large deck of cards. • Requires less fine motor control.
Deal or discard cards at a specific target a specified distance away. • Requires more proximal and distal strength. • Requires more proximal and distal motor control.	Place cards in front of client. • Requires less proximal and distal strength. • Requires less proximal and distal motor control.
Set deck on table rather than in unaffected hand, and grasp top card with affected hand. • Requires more pinch grip.	Use unaffected hand to hold the deck and slide the top card over for affected hand to grasp. • Requires less pinch grip.

Task Mastery:
1. Consistently deals or discards card at specified distance.
2. Consistently grasps card on first attempt.

Ideas for related tasks	Rationale
Filing papers	Requires pinch grip. Requires proximal and distal motor control.
Counting money	Requires pinch grip. Requires proximal and distal motor control.

90. Task: Bowling

Key Impairments Addressed:
1. Decreased proximal strength
2. Decreased distal strength
3. Decreased proximal motor control
4. Decreased distal motor control

Materials:
Bowling ball or lighter weight ball similar in size
Hallway or outdoor space
Bowling pins or other target

Task Description:
1. Grasp ball with bilateral hands, and place fingers of affected hand into holes.
2. Bowl down a hallway or outdoor space.

Grading Task:

Increase difficulty	Decrease difficulty
Use heavy bowling ball.	Use lightweight bowling ball.
• Requires more proximal and distal strength.	• Requires less proximal and distal strength.
Place pins at end of long hallway or sidewalk.	Place pins in close proximity to client.
• Requires more proximal and distal motor control.	• Requires less proximal and distal motor control.

Task Mastery:
1. Consistently grasps ball and rolls it toward targets without dropping.

Ideas for related tasks	Rationale
Swinging tennis racquet	Requires proximal and distal strength. Requires proximal distal motor control.
Throwing a horseshoe	Requires proximal and distal strength. Requires proximal and distal motor control.

91. Task: Placing DVD into DVD player

Key Impairments Addressed:
1. Decreased distal strength
2. Decreased pinch grip
3. Decreased distal motor control

Materials:
DVD
DVD player

Task Description:
1. Open DVD case with bilateral hands.
2. Grasp DVD with affected hand and place in DVD player.
3. Remove from DVD player with affected hand and return to case.
4. Close case with bilateral hands.

Grading Task:

Increase difficulty	Decrease difficulty
Place DVD player on elevated shelf.	Place DVD player on low shelf.
• Requires more proximal strength.	• Requires less proximal strength.
Place DVD case in organizer.	Set DVD case on table.
• Requires more distal strength and motor control.	• Requires less distal strength and motor control.

Task Mastery:
1. Grasps DVD on first attempt and places into player without dropping.
2. Places DVD back into case on first attempt.

Idea for related task	Rationale
Placing CD into CD player	Requires distal strength and motor control. Requires pinch grip.

92. Task: Turning pages of book

Key Impairments Addressed:
1. Decreased distal strength
2. Decreased pinch grip
3. Decreased fine motor control

Materials:
Book

Task Description:
1. Hold book with unaffected upper extremity, and turn pages with affected hand.

Grading Task:

Increase difficulty	Decrease difficulty
Use newspaper or magazine with thin pages. • Requires more pinch grip.	Use book with thick pages (i.e., children's board book). • Requires less pinch grip.
Place book on table. • Requires more proximal strength and pinch grip. • Requires proximal motor control.	Place book on lap. • Requires less proximal strength.
Have client turn to a certain page number. • Requires more fine motor control.	Allow client to flip any number of pages over. • Requires less fine motor control.

Task Mastery:
1. Consistently grasps and turns appropriate number of pages.
2. Consistently turns page on first attempt.

Ideas for related tasks	Rationale
Flipping through mail	Requires pinch grip and distal motor control.
Opening greeting card	Requires distal strength and pinch grip.
Flipping through newspaper	Requires distal strength and pinch grip.

93. Task: Playing Connect Four

Key Impairments Addressed:
1. Decreased proximal strength
2. Decreased pinch grip
3. Decreased proximal motor control

Materials:
Connect Four game

Task Description:
1. Grasp game piece, and place into slot of game grid.

Grading Task:

Increase difficulty	Decrease difficulty
Place grid at arm's length from client. • Requires more proximal strength and motor control.	Place grid close to client. • Requires less proximal strength and motor control.
Place game pieces in small cup. • Requires more fine motor control.	Place game pieces in pile on table. • Requires less fine motor control.
	Place game grid on nonslip material to prevent slipping. • Requires less proximal motor control.

Task Mastery:
1. Consistently grasps game piece on first attempt.
2. Places game piece into slot without dropping.

Ideas for related tasks	Rationale
Playing board games	Requires pinch grip. Requires proximal and distal motor control.
Sorting coins	Requires pinch grip. Requires proximal and distal motor control.
Placing coin in coin bank	Requires pinch grip. Requires proximal and distal motor control.

Task: Threading beads onto necklace

Key Impairments Addressed:
1. Decreased pinch grip
2. Decreased fine motor control

Materials:
String
Beads of various sizes

Task Description:
1. Grasp bead with affected hand.
2. Thread onto string held in unaffected hand.

Grading Task:

Increase difficulty	Decrease difficulty
Use small beads. • Requires more fine motor control.	Use large beads. • Requires less fine motor control.
Use beads with a small bead-hole-to-string circumference ratio. • Requires more fine motor control.	Use large bead-hole-to-string circumference ratio. • Requires less fine motor control.
Retrieve beads from small dish. • Requires more fine motor control.	Retrieve beads from large pile on table. • Requires less fine motor control.
Retrieve specific size, shape, or color of bead from dish containing various sizes, shapes, and colors. • Requires more fine motor control.	Retrieve any kind of bead. • Requires less fine motor control.

Task Mastery:
1. Consistently grasps bead on first attempt.
2. Threads bead on string without dropping.

Idea for related task	Rationale
Sewing	Requires pinch grip. Requires fine motor control.

95. Task: Playing bingo

Key Impairments Addressed:
1. Decreased pinch grip
2. Decreased fine motor control

Materials:
Bingo card
Bingo markers (or other small item)

Task Description:
1. Practitioner calls out bingo number.
2. Affected hand grasps marker and places it on appropriate spot on card.
3. Hand returns to table.

Grading Task:

Increase difficulty	Decrease difficulty
Use small marker. • Requires more fine motor control.	Use large marker. • Requires less fine motor control.
Hold markers in affected palm and transfer one by one to fingertips. • Requires more fine motor control.	Pick up markers from table. • Requires less fine motor control.
Place bingo card further away from client. • Requires more proximal strength and motor control.	Place bingo card close to client. • Requires less proximal strength and motor control.

Task Mastery:
1. Consistently grasps marker on first attempt.
2. Consistently places on card on first attempt.
3. Demonstrates controlled reaching.

Ideas for related tasks	Rationale
Playing Connect Four	Requires proximal strength. Requires pinch grip and fine motor control.
Playing board game	Requires pinch grip and fine motor control.
Placing pills in pill sorter	Requires pinch grip and fine motor control.

96. Task: Swinging tennis racquet

Key Impairments Addressed:
1. Decreased proximal strength
2. Decreased distal strength
3. Decreased proximal motor control
4. Decreased distal motor control

Materials:
Tennis racquet

Task Description:
1. Hold tennis racquet with affected hand and swing at a ball that practitioner tosses toward client.
2. Practitioner retrieves ball and repeats.

Grading Task:

Increase difficulty	Decrease difficulty
Toss a tennis ball before swinging. • Requires more proximal and distal motor control.	Toss a balloon before swinging. • Requires less proximal and distal motor control.
Use various types of swings (e.g., backhand, forehand, overhead). • Requires more proximal strength. • Requires more proximal and distal motor control.	Allow client to select how he or she swings. • Requires less proximal and distal motor control.

Task Mastery:
1. Consistently makes contact with ball on each swing.
2. Swings with desired accuracy and using desired type of swing.

Ideas for related tasks	Rationale
Swinging a golf club	Requires proximal and distal strength. Requires proximal and distal motor control.
Throwing a ball	Requires proximal and distal strength. Requires proximal and distal motor control.
Bowling	Requires proximal and distal strength. Requires proximal and distal motor control.

97. Task: Planting flowers

Key Impairments Addressed:
1. Decreased proximal strength
2. Decreased distal strength
3. Decreased distal motor control

Materials:
Topsoil or rice
Trowel
Flowerpot
Flowers

Task Description:
1. Grasp trowel with affected hand and scoop soil or rice.
2. Dump into flower pot.
3. Grasp flowers and place into pot.
4. Use bilateral hands to pack soil or rice into pot.

Grading Task:

Increase difficulty	Decrease difficulty
Use a heavy trowel. • Requires more grip strength.	Use a lightweight trowel. • Requires less grip strength.
Use packed soil. • Requires more distal strength.	Use small amount of loose soil. • Requires less distal strength.
	Use a trowel with a built-up handle. • Requires less distal strength and motor control.

Task Mastery:
1. Consistently grasps trowel on first attempt.
2. Demonstrates control while scooping soil and dumping into pot.
3. Does not spill soil on table.

Ideas for related tasks	Rationale
Kneading dough	Requires distal strength.
Scooping sugar into bowl	Requires distal strength and motor control.

98. Task: Golfing

Key Impairments Addressed:
1. Decreased distal strength
2. Decreased grip strength
3. Decreased proximal motor control

Materials:
Golf club (putter recommended if indoors or in small area)
Ball (plastic toy ball suggested)
Hole or other target for ball
Long hallway (optional)

Task Description:
1. Grip club to prepare for swing.
2. Hit or putt golf ball.

Grading Task:

Increase difficulty	Decrease difficulty
Hit ball a long distance. • Requires more proximal motor control.	Place target a few feet from ball. • Requires less proximal motor control.
Use small ball. • Requires more proximal motor control during swing.	Use large ball. • Requires less proximal motor control during swing.
Hit ball toward small target (i.e., small bucket tipped on its side). • Requires more proximal motor control.	Hit ball toward large target (i.e., large towel on the floor over which the ball must roll). • Requires less proximal motor control.

Task Mastery:
1. Consistently hits ball on first attempt.
2. Consistently reaches target.
3. Demonstrates smooth trajectory of movement during swing.

Ideas for related tasks	Rationale
Sweeping floor	Requires proximal and distal strength. Requires proximal motor control.
Swinging tennis racquet	Requires proximal and distal strength. Requires proximal motor control.

99. Task: Lighting candle

Key Impairments Addressed:
1. Decreased distal strength
2. Decreased pinch grip
3. Decreased fine motor control

Materials:
Matches (use substitute for safety)
Matchbook (use substitute for safety)
or
Lighter (without lighter fluid, or keep safety lock on)

Task Description:
1. Grasp match with affected hand and simulate striking against matchbook; light candle.
or
2. Grasp lighter with affected hand and simulate lighting candle.

Grading Task:

Increase difficulty	Decrease difficulty
Use small match and matchbook.	Use large match and matchbook.
• Requires more fine motor control.	• Requires less fine motor control.
Use hand-held lighter.	Use long-reach candle lighter.
• Requires more distal strength.	• Requires less distal strength.

Task Mastery:
1. Consistently grasps match and strikes cleanly on first attempt.
2. Consistently presses button and makes contact with candle on first attempt.

Ideas for related tasks	Rationale
Locking deadbolt	Requires pinch grip.
Turning pages in book	Requires fine motor control.
	Requires distal strength.

100. Task: Taking photo

Key Impairments Addressed:
1. Decreased proximal strength
2. Decreased distal strength
3. Decreased distal motor control

Materials:
Camera

Task Description:
1. Grasps camera with affected hand.
2. Snaps photo with finger of affected hand.

Grading Task:

Increase difficulty	Decrease difficulty
Use camera with small or stiff button.	Use camera with large button, such as a toy camera.
• Requires more distal motor control.	• Requires less distal motor control.
Use heavy-duty camera.	Use lightweight camera.
• Requires more proximal strength.	• Requires less proximal strength.

Task Mastery:
1. Consistently presses button to take photo on first attempt.

Ideas for related tasks	Rationale
Pressing power button on television	Requires distal strength and motor control.
Powering on a cell phone	Requires distal strength and motor control.

Exhibit 4.6. Blank Task Description Form

Task: _____

Key Impairments Addressed:

1. _____
2. _____
3. _____

Materials:

_____
_____

Task Description:

1. _____
2. _____
3. _____
4. _____

Grading Task:

Increase difficulty	Decrease difficulty

Task Mastery:

1. _____
2. _____

Ideas for related tasks	Rationale

CHAPTER 5

Planning and Organizing Tasks Into a Treatment Program

The initial evaluation is complete, and goals and tasks have been selected; it is now time to transform the tasks into a treatment program to maximize function and performance in daily life. Several considerations arise in determining a treatment program.

Length and Frequency of Treatment Programs

Typically, treatment sessions in clinical settings last 45 minutes to 1 hour, and the tasks in this manual were created with this timeframe in mind. To maximize treatment time and minimize boredom during a session, consider selecting 2–3 tasks per session, which will allow ample time to work on each task so that a high number of repetitions are attainable. Try to perform the same tasks on a daily basis for at least 2 weeks (see Chapter 6, "Task-Specific Training as the Home Exercise Program," for ways to increase therapy time outside of formal therapy sessions). During this time, tasks should be graded continually to achieve optimal outcomes. If after 2 weeks, improvement is minimal to none, switch to another meaningful task that may be more beneficial to practice.

Selecting Complementary Tasks to Practice in a Program

Treatment sessions should consist of a variety of tasks that target different movements. Upper-extremity (UE) movements are often thought of in terms of gross motor and fine motor control, and clinicians may be tempted to select tasks that work solely on one or the other. Because many daily activities involve gross motor control, fine motor control, and bilateral activities, it is important not to concentrate on only one of these areas during a session. In other words, do not select 3 activities that aim to improve only gross motor control (i.e., unilateral shoulder flexion tasks such as lifting cans onto a cabinet shelf, applying paint to a wall using

a roller, and unloading a dishwasher). Instead, select 3 tasks that complement each other. For instance, the task of lifting cans onto a cabinet shelf could be paired with picking up a laundry basket to work on a bilateral task and opening containers to include a fine motor component in the treatment program. Naturally, evaluation results will lead to the impairments that most affect the client's participation in functional tasks, so the movement focus will be different for each client.

Many daily activities require the use of both arms for full participation, and during the day, people spend equal amounts of time using both UEs (Bailey & Lang, in press). Activities such as putting on a shirt, tying shoes, and unloading the dishwasher are just a few of the common activities that people do on a consistent basis that require the use of both arms. Many of the tasks included in this manual take this fact into consideration and were created to encourage bilateral use of the UEs during daily activities. When developing a treatment program, consider selecting at least 1 task that is bilateral in nature. Incorporating the affected UE into a functional task that is bilateral in nature may provide an opportunity for clients with less residual movement to become more independent in performing daily activities. At some point during treatment, it will be necessary to decide whether the affected arm will be the dexterous one or the supportive one (i.e., used as a gross assist) in a task. Bilateral tasks also allow practice for the supportive arm and may ultimately lead to improved function.

Treatment programs need to take into consideration each client's unique needs. For instance, Figures 3.1 to 3.3 addressed how to select goals for clients with limited, moderate, and higher UE function. Case Examples 5.1 to 5.3 discuss each of the examples from Chapter 3, "Task-Specific Training," with respect to constructing an individualized task-specific training program.

Case Example 5.1. Limited Upper-Extremity Function

Assessment scores indicated that a client with limited movement had no ability to fractionate (individuate) finger movement, minimal gross motor movement, and greatly increased muscle tone affecting the ability to move. This client was also 6 months poststroke. His selected goals were (1) using tools, (2) drinking from a cup, (3) incorporating the affected arm into eating tasks, (4) turning a doorknob, and (5) stabilizing paper during handwriting tasks. Given the client's history, he was not likely to regain a lot more movement. We therefore selected tasks that focused on gross movement of the affected arm (i.e., stabilizing a bucket for digging, opening a door handle, turning off a light switch, lifting a laundry basket, wiping down a table, and grasping utensils). In this scenario, the client always performed 1–2 tasks that were bilateral in nature as well as tasks that used gross motor versus fine motor control.

Treatment Program Adaptation for People With Pain

Shoulder pain is common after stroke (Lindgren, Jonsson, Norrving, & Lindgren, 2007). People experiencing shoulder pain may be limited in their ability to participate in rehabilitation, resulting in poor outcomes (Roy, Sands, & Hill, 1994; Roy, Sands, Hill, Harrison, & Marshall, 1995; Turner-Stokes & Jackson, 2002; Wanklyn, Forster, & Young, 1996). In addition, many people have other aches and pains in various body parts that often have been present for years. Task-specific training programs should not increase the pain a person experiences. The way tasks are implemented can be adjusted to avoid painful movements. For example, if a client with shoulder pain and mild subluxation tends to abduct his shoulder while reaching up to paint a wall, eliciting pain, the client can be encouraged to avoid painful motions by painting in a diagonal motion, adducting the shoulder, or by limiting the range through which he elevates his shoulder. In a case such as this one, shoulder taping to address subluxation may be indicated.

If pain is a concern, it should be monitored and documented regularly (see Exhibit 3.3 in Chapter 3, "Task-Specific Training"). One process we have adopted is to ask the client to rate his or her pain (on a visual analog scale or numeric rating scale) before a treatment session and then after the treatment session. This rating allows us to see whether pain has increased since the client was last seen in therapy and whether the therapy session inadvertently increased the pain. Interestingly, we have often seen reports of pain de-

cline by the end of a session (Birkenmeier et al., 2010). This process could be readily implemented in routine clinical care.

Treatment Program Adaptations for People With Ataxia, Apraxia, and Hemispatial Neglect

The tasks in this manual are not specifically designed to address ataxia, apraxia, or hemispatial neglect. It is inevitable, however, that clients with these additional impairments will appear on a clinician's caseload.

Ataxia

Ataxia results from damage to the cerebellum or its input and output structures. The term *ataxia* may be applied to specific movements such as ataxic reach or ataxic gait. It means that movements are spatially and temporally uncoordinated and is used in a more general sense to describe poor coordination and inaccurate and variable movements (Sathian et al., 2011). UE ataxia can be observed during execution of a task, such as reaching or grasping (Bastian, 1997). A client with ataxic movement may demonstrate decreased accuracy and speed of movement, errors in acceleration and deceleration, and tremor or oscillations of limb segments (Morton & Bastian, 2009). A task may be set up to control or limit the amount of ataxia interfering with movement execution.

Some suggestions for setting up a task to address ataxia include

- Stabilize the proximal UE segment to control the degrees of freedom of movement allowed.

Case Example 5.2. Moderate Upper-Extremity Function

For a client with moderate arm function after stroke, we selected more whole tasks. Assessment results indicated that the client had some grasp, pinch, and gross motor movement, plus a small increase in muscle tone that was not affecting movement. The client's selected goals were (1) reaching to tuck a shirt in behind the back, (2) reaching across the body to adjust a collar, (3) combing hair, (4) reaching into cabinets, and (5) picking up and maintaining grasp on a variety of objects. Treatment tasks included tucking in a shirt, folding down a shirt collar, picking up pens and placing them in a pencil holder, drying pots and pans, combing hair, typing, throwing a basketball, and pouring juice into a cup. In this situation, a variety of bilateral tasks were selected in addition to tasks addressing both gross motor and fine motor control. The likelihood of the client's being able to use the affected arm functionally was much higher than that of the client with limited UE function. For this reason, selecting some tasks that used the arm as a stabilizer and some tasks that encouraged full functional use of the arm was reasonable.

For example, a client may rest his or her elbow on the table while reaching for a fork or rest the forearm against his or her trunk while opening a jar.

- Limit the range of motion through which the client must move the segment. Placing the fork closer to the client or lowering the shelf from which to grasp the jar may allow the client to complete the task with fewer errors.
- Encourage the client to move slowly during execution of the movement. A faster movement, with high acceleration, may result in less precision and more errors than a slower movement.

Apraxia

Apraxia is the inability to perform skilled, purposeful movements, often with a limb that has adequate strength and sensation (Sathian et al., 2011; Wheaton & Hallett, 2007). It can be considered a cognitive problem that results in an impaired ability to program motor systems to perform purposeful skilled movements (Heilman, Rothi, & Valenstein, 1982). UE apraxia can be observed during execution of skilled actions, particularly ones that require a sequence of movements and interaction with objects. It often appears that the person with apraxia does not know how to complete the task and interact with the object.

There are different subtypes of apraxia, and comprehensive standardized testing can determine the subtype and lead to suggestions for treatment. Although the treatment tasks provided in this manual do not directly address apraxia, a clinician can do several things in a treatment session to minimize the influence of apraxia on the training.

Some suggestions for setting up a task to address apraxia include

- Focus on the specific task and how the task is performed at home. Perform the task in the least complex manner that corresponds with how the task is performed at home.
- Perform tasks that involve simple movements (1- or 2-step tasks instead of 3- to 4-step tasks).
- Do not change tasks too frequently. Allow the client ample time to practice tasks and become proficient before switching to new tasks.

Hemispatial Neglect

Hemispatial neglect is another cognitive impairment that may interfere with the execution of movement and limit daily participation in desired activities (Appelros, Karlsson, Seiger, & Nydevik, 2002, 2003; Appelros, Nydevik, Karlsson, Thorwalls, & Seiger, 2004; Buxbaum et al., 2004). As with apraxia, neglect has different subtypes such that a person may have motor, body, or visual neglect. The fundamental impairment of neglect is the inability to attend and respond to stimuli, often on the left side of the body (Corbetta et al., 2005). Observation of a person with neglect can lead one to think that the person has more severe paresis and greater loss of somatosensation than the impairment results indicate. Several modifications to task-specific training can be implemented with clients experiencing unilateral neglect.

Some suggestions for setting up a task to address unilateral neglect include

- Force the use of the neglected side of the body. For example, if the task of washing and drying dishes is selected, place all of the task materials (e.g., towel, dishes) on the neglected side of the body.
- Choose at least 1 task that is bilateral in nature. Select an activity that would be difficult to perform without the use of both arms. For example, tying shoes is unlikely to be successful if the client does not use both hands to perform the task.

- Provide visual cues, verbal cues, or both to direct attention to the neglected side of the body. These cues can include using a mirror to allow the client to observe the task he or she is performing or using colored tape on the table so the client knows that he or she must look for the tape.

Summary

When planning and organizing tasks into a treatment plan, it is important to consider the treatment program's length and frequency, appropriately selecting complementary tasks and adapting programs for clients with pain or ataxia, apraxia, and hemispatial neglect.

CHAPTER 6

Task-Specific Training as the Home Exercise Program

Growing trends in health care delivery include decreased lengths of stay in the hospital system as well as fewer visits for outpatient services (Coupar, Pollock, Legg, Sackley, & van Vliet, 2012; Fearon & Langhorne, 2012). The result for people post stroke is less time spent with rehabilitation professionals. Continued efforts to make stroke service delivery effective and efficient have caused growth in home-based care and increased use of home exercise programs.

Home exercise programs are tasks prescribed by a health care professional that are carried out in a client's home. Traditionally, home exercise programs are thought of as strictly therapeutic exercise (e.g., upper-extremity strengthening, stretching). As discussed previously, tasks must be practiced to improve performance.

Task-specific training is repetitive practice of functional activities, not therapeutic exercise, and this training can be applied to a client's home exercise program. In addition, achieving mastery of a skill or maintaining a current ability requires additional work outside of traditional rehabilitation services. It is up to the client to carry through with the home exercise program. Certain characteristics should be considered when prescribing a home exercise program: type and difficulty of task, number of tasks, and participation. Sample and blank home exercise programs are provided in Exhibits 6.1 and 6.2.

Type and Difficulty of Tasks

Type of task is an essential part of a home exercise program. A task should be meaningful to the person, address key impairments and functional limitations, and be at an appropriate level of difficulty. People are more likely to complete tasks if they are intrinsically important (Leach et al., 2010; Rebeiro & Polgar, 1999). For example, if a client has the goal to improve handwriting, the client may be more adherent to the home

exercise program if he or she practices a task such as signing a check or receipt with his or her name versus copying text from a book. The task of signing a check or receipt is personal to the client and a task he or she may actually perform each day outside of therapy.

In addition, the task should be specific to the impairment or the limitation that is being addressed (Kleim & Jones, 2008). To improve casting with a reel rod for fishing, casting must be practiced, not tying on a lure. Finally, tasks should be graded to match the client's motor capabilities—the just-right challenge. Refer to Chapter 3, "Task-Specific Training," for in-depth guidance on increasing or decreasing the difficulty of tasks and Chapter 4, "Toolbox of Upper-Extremity Tasks," for specific tasks.

Number of Tasks

Just as the type and difficulty of a task are important to consider, practitioners must also balance the number of tasks prescribed, including the total time required for home exercise program completion. A total of 3–5 tasks with 2 or 3 performed daily is typical in a home exercise program. With fewer than 3, a client may become bored. It is also challenging to address several impairments with only 1–2 tasks. Conversely, prescribing more than five tasks may overwhelm the client and result in limited task practice. Even with written instruction and pictures, it can be challenging to recall how to perform a task correctly. Thus, the more tasks that are prescribed, the greater the likelihood that 1 or more of them will be performed incorrectly or not at all.

Clinicians must consider not only the time required to complete a task but also the summative time commitment. People may be more willing to finish or more able to fit in a program that takes 20–30 minutes rather than 60–70 minutes. In addition, if a client performs so many repetitions of a task that he or she is

Exhibit 6.1. Sample Home Exercise Program

Name:_____   Date:_____

Goals:

1. Improve independence with washing the arm and underarm.
2. Decrease time to tie shoes using both hands.
3. Play cards with bridge group.

Tasks:

1. Washing body to improve shoulder and elbow motion and strength and to improve grip
   Complete 50 repetitions 1/day (approximately 10 minutes)

   Materials: Wash cloth or bath mitt.

   Task description (1 repetition): Stand at table with washcloth on table; grasp cloth with the right hand and wash the left arm from the hand up to the shoulder and armpit and back down; replace washcloth on table and let go.

   If the task becomes too easy, try one of the following:
   ☐ Placing the cloth on a shelf instead of the table
   ☐ Using a hand towel.

2. Tying shoes to improve finger control and strength
   Complete 15 repetitions 1/day (approximately 10 minutes)

   Materials: Tennis shoe with laces.

   Task description (1 repetition): Sit in chair holding shoe between thighs; grasp laces with both hands; cross laces and tighten; tie a bow and tighten; untie laces.

   If the task becomes too easy, try one of the following:
   ☐ Using smaller or thinner laces
   ☐ Tying and double-knotting laces.

3. **Playing cards** to improve shoulder and elbow motion and strength and to improve grip
   Complete 50 repetitions 1/day (approximately 10 minutes)

   Materials: Deck of playing cards; optional: partner.

   Task description (1 repetition): Sit at table holding cards in the left hand; grasp card with the right hand and place on table or hand to partner (face side up).

   If the task becomes too easy, try one of the following:
   ☐ Using a smaller deck of cards
   ☐ Playing bridge.

Remember to be safe and to stop if the activity becomes painful.
Questions? Contact clinician at (XXX) XXX-XXXX.

Exhibit 6.2. Blank Home Exercise Program Form

Name:_____   Date:_____

Goals:

1.
2.
3.
4.

Tasks:

1.

   Complete repetitions __/day (approximately __ minutes)

   Materials:

   Task description (1 repetition):

   If the task becomes too easy, try one of the following:
   ☐
   ☐

2.

   Complete repetitions __/day (approximately __ minutes)

   Materials:

   Task description (1 repetition):

   If the task becomes too easy, try one of the following:
   ☐
   ☐

3.

   Complete repetitions __/day (approximately __ minutes)

   Materials:

   Task description (1 repetition):

   If the task becomes too easy, try one of the following:
   ☐
   ☐

Remember to be safe and to stop if the activity becomes painful.
Questions? Contact clinician at (___) ___-____.

fatigued and cannot participate in daily activities, the client may choose not to complete the home exercise program at all.

Adherence to a home exercise program is a common challenge (Simek, McPhate, & Haines, 2012; Spink et al., 2011), and clinicians may need to experiment and continuously follow up with clients to get the right exercise prescription for each of them.

Participation in the Home Exercise Program

The final and arguably most important issue that should be considered when prescribing a home exercise program is the likelihood of participation. A client's participation depends on both his or her cognitive ability to understand and execute the task and his or her willingness to participate. If a client has severe cognitive deficits, he or she will not be able to understand and perform an independent home exercise program. The client will likely need a caregiver to provide instruction and to assist with task completion. If the client is able to understand the task, it is important that the clinician educate the client on how it addresses the client's personal goals and fits into the overall plan of care.

A critical ingredient for success is providing the client with a sense of autonomy and encouraging the client's active participation in his or her own care. Asking the client to keep a log of task completion is a useful strategy that allows him or her to take responsibility for treatment and allows the client and clinician to track progress (Yuen et al., 2013). An example log is provided in Exhibit 6.3. If a client is unwilling to adhere to the home exercise program, the tasks will not be completed. In these instances, it is important to explain to the client and caregiver the role of the home exercise program within the plan of care and to work through any barriers that might be hindering program completion. If the client or caregiver is unwilling or unable to complete the program, changes to goals, treatment, and plan of care will ultimately need to occur.

Although we have used the term *home exercise program* throughout this chapter, it is important to note that home is not the only place for additional practice. Several studies have shown that, during acute care and inpatient rehabilitation stays, people after stroke spend the majority of time alone and in bed (Bernhardt, Chan, Nicola, & Collier, 2007; Bernhardt, Dewey, Thrift, & Donnan, 2004; Lang et al., 2009). Taking advantage of the time available to people when they are in the hospital, an inpatient rehabilitation facility, or a skilled nursing facility will allow for increased practice time and maximized treatment.

A challenge commonly faced with home exercise programs is that they are done at home and not under the direct supervision of a health care professional. For these reasons, falls and overuse injuries are valid concerns. It is critical that the practitioner design the task to be challenging for the client yet safe enough for him or her to do alone or with the supervision of a caregiver. To achieve this goal, the practitioner must give explicit directions. See Exhibit 6.1 for a sample home exercise program and the type of directions provided. Examples of how to make tasks safer would be to have the person sit or stand while holding onto the counter, keep items close by, have a caregiver supervise, monitor for pain or fatigue, and take rest breaks as needed.

Suggestions for maximizing practice through a home exercise program while the client is away from home include

- Educate the client, family member, or both on tasks that the client can do in the evening.
- Provide a kit with the necessary materials in the client's room (i.e., a plastic tote that contains a pot and spoon if the client is working on stirring). For tasks such as hair brushing or turning a TV remote on and off, a kit may not be necessary.
- Request that the client, family member, or nurse track dosage (i.e., time, repetitions) on a log. This log will help the practitioner determine when it may be time to upgrade or downgrade a task.

Summary

After stroke, people are spending less time with rehabilitation professionals, contributing to growth in home-based care. Task-specific training can be applied to a client's home exercise program. Practitioners should consider characteristics such as type and difficulty of task, number of tasks, and participation when prescribing a home exercise program.

Exhibit 6.3. Home Exercise Program Tracking Log

Date	Repetitions	Time	Repetitions	Time	Repetitions	Time
Task 1						
Task 2						
Task 3						
Task 4						
Task 5						
Total						

References

Adkins, D. L., Boychuk, J., Remple, M. S., & Kleim, J. A. (2006). Motor training induces experience-specific patterns of plasticity across motor cortex and spinal cord. *Journal of Applied Physiology, 101,* 1776–1782. http://dx.doi.org/10.1152/japplphysiol.00515.2006

Appelros, P., Karlsson, G. M., Seiger, A., & Nydevik, I. (2002). Neglect and anosognosia after first-ever stroke: Incidence and relationship to disability. *Journal of Rehabilitation Medicine, 34,* 215–220.

Appelros, P., Karlsson, G. M., Seiger, A., & Nydevik, I. (2003). Prognosis for patients with neglect and anosognosia with special reference to cognitive impairment. *Journal of Rehabilitation Medicine, 35,* 254–248.

Appelros, P., Nydevik, I., Karlsson, G. M., Thorwalls, A., & Seiger, A. (2004). Recovery from unilateral neglect after right-hemisphere stroke. *Disability and Rehabilitation, 26,* 471–477.

Bailey, R. R., & Lang, C. E. (in press). Upper extremity activity in adults: Referent values using accelerometry. *Journal of Rehabilitation Research and Development.*

Barreca, S., Gowland, C. K., Stratford, P., Huijbregts, M., Griffiths, J., Torresin, W., . . . Masters, L. (2004). Development of the Chedoke Arm and Hand Activity Inventory: Theoretical constructs, item generation, and selection. *Topics in Stroke Rehabilitation, 11,* 31–42.

Barreca, S. R., Stratford, P. W., Lambert, C. L., Masters, L. M., & Streiner, D. L. (2005). Test–retest reliability, validity, and sensitivity of the Chedoke Arm and Hand Activity Inventory: A new measure of upper-limb function for survivors of stroke. *Archives of Physical and Medical Rehabilitation, 86,* 1616–1622. http://dx.doi.org/10.1016/j.apmr.2005.03.017

Barreca, S., Stratford, P., Masters, L., Lambert, C. L., Griffiths, J., & McBay, C. (2006). Validation of three shortened versions of the Chedoke Arm and Hand Activity Inventory. *Physiotherapy Canada, 58,* 1–9. http://dx.doi.org/10.3138/ptc.58.2.148

Barry, J. G., Ross, S. A., & Woehrle, J. (2012). Therapy incorporating a dynamic wrist–hand orthosis versus manual assistance in chronic stroke: A pilot study. *Journal of Neurological Physical Therapy, 36,* 17–24. http://dx.doi.org/10.1097/NPT.0b013e318246203e

Bastian, A. J. (1997). Mechanisms of ataxia. *Physical Therapy, 77,* 672–675.

Bayona, N. A., Bitensky, J., Salter, K., & Teasell, R. (2005). The role of task-specific training in rehabilitation therapies. *Topics in Stroke Rehabilitation, 12,* 58–65.

Beebe, J. A., & Lang, C. E. (2008). Absence of a proximal to distal gradient of motor deficits in the upper extremity early after stroke. *Clinical Neurophysiology, 119,* 2074–2085. http://dx.doi.org/10.1016/j.clinph.2008.04.293

Beebe, J. A., & Lang, C. E. (2009a). Active range of motion predicts upper extremity function 3 months after stroke. *Stroke, 40,* 1772–1779. http://dx.doi.org/10.1161/STROKEAHA.108.536763

Beebe, J. A., & Lang, C. E. (2009b). Relationships and responsiveness of six upper extremity function tests during the first six months of recovery after stroke. *Journal of Neurological Physical Therapy, 33,* 96–103. http://dx.doi.org/10.1097/NPT.0b013e3181a33638

Bernhardt, J., Chan, J. Nicola, I., & Collier, J. M. (2007). Little therapy, little physical activity: Rehabilitation within the first 14 days of organized stroke unit care. *Journal of Rehabilitation Medicine, 39,* 43–48. http://dx.doi.org/10.2340/16501977-0013

Bernhardt, J., Dewey, H., Thrift, A., & Donnan, G. (2004). Inactive and alone: Physical activity within the first 14 days of acute stroke unit care. *Stroke, 35,* 1005–1009. http://dx.doi.org/10.1161/01.STR.0000120727.40792.40

Birkenmeier, R. L., Prager, E. M., & Lang, C. E. (2010). Translating animal doses of task-specific training to people with chronic stroke in 1-hour therapy sessions: A proof-of-concept study. *Neurorehabilitation and Neural Repair, 24,* 620–635. http://dx.doi.org/10.1177/1545968310361957

Bland, M. D., Sturmoski, A., Whitson, M., Harris, H., Connor, L. T., Fucetola, R., . . . Lang, C. E. (2013). Clinician adherence to a standardized assessment battery across settings and disciplines in a poststroke rehabilitation population. *Archives of Physical Medicine and Reha-*

bilitation, 94, 1048–1053. http://dx.doi.org/10.1016/j.apmr.2013.02.004

Bohannon, R. W., & Smith, M. B. (1987a). Interrater reliability of a modified Ashworth scale of muscle spasticity. *Physical Therapy, 67,* 206–207.

Bohannon, R. W., & Smith, M. B. (1987b). Upper extremity strength deficits in hemiplegic stroke patients: Relationship between admission and discharge assessment and time since onset. *Archives of Physical Medicine and Rehabilitation, 68,* 155–157.

Boyd, L., & Winstein, C. (2006). Explicit information interferes with implicit motor learning of both continuous and discrete movement tasks after stroke. *Journal of Neurological Physical Therapy, 30,* 46–57; discussion 58–59.

Buxbaum, L. J., Ferraro, M. K., Veramonti, T., Farne, A., Whyte, J., Ladavas, E., . . . Coslett, H. B. (2004). Hemispatial neglect: Subtypes, neuroanatomy, and disability. *Neurology, 62,* 749–756.

Carey, J. R., Anderson, K. M., Kimberley, T. J., Lewis, S. M., Auerbach, E. J., & Ugurbil, K. (2004). fMRI analysis of ankle movement tracking training in subject with stroke. *Experimental Brain Research, 154,* 281–290. http://dx.doi.org/10.1007/s00221-003-1662-7

Carey, J. R., Kimberley, T. J., Lewis, S. M., Auerbach, E. J., Dorsey, L., Rundquist, P., & Ugurbil, K. (2002). Analysis of fMRI and finger tracking training in subjects with chronic stroke. *Brain, 125,* 773–788. http://dx.doi.org/10.1093/brain/awf091

Carmichael, S. T. (2008). Themes and strategies for studying the biology of stroke recovery in the poststroke epoch. *Stroke, 39,* 1380–1388. http://dx.doi.org/10.1161/STROKEAHA.107.499962

Carter, A. R., Shulman, G. L., & Corbetta, M. (2012). Why use a connectivity-based approach to study stroke and recovery of function? *Neuroimage, 62,* 2271–2280. http://dx.doi.org/10.1016/j.neuroimage.2012.02.070

Collin, C., & Wade, D. (1990). Assessing motor impairment after stroke: A pilot reliability study. *Journal of Neurology, Neurosurgery and Psychiatry 53,* 576–579. http://dx.doi.org/10.1016/j.neuroimage.2012.02.070

Connell, L. A., & Tyson, S. F. (2012). Clinical reality of measuring upper-limb ability in neurologic conditions: A systematic review. *Archives of Physical Medicine and Rehabilitation, 93,* 221–228. http://dx.doi.org/10.1016/j.apmr.2011.09.015

Corbetta, M., Kincade, M. J., Lewis, C., Snyder, A. Z., & Sapir, A. (2005). Neural basis and recovery of spatial attention deficits in spatial neglect. *Nature Neuroscience, 8,* 1603–1610. http://dx.doi.org/10.1038/nn1574

Coupar, F., Pollock, A., Legg, L. A., Sackley, C., & van Vliet, P. (2012). Home-based therapy programmes for upper limb functional recovery following stroke. *Cochrane Database of Systematic Reviews, 2012*(5), CD006755. http://dx.doi.org/10.1002/14651858.CD006755.pub2

Cup, E. H., Scholte op Reimer, W. J., Thijssen, M. C., & van Kuyk-Minis, M. A. (2003). Reliability and validity of the Canadian Occupational Performance Measure in stroke patients. *Clinical Rehabilitation, 17,* 402–409. http://dx.doi.org/10.1191/0269215503cr635oa

Dedding, C., Cardol, M., Eyssen, I. C., Dekker, J., & Beelen, A. (2004). Validity of the Canadian Occupational Performance Measure: A client-centred outcome measurement. *Clinical Rehabilitation, 18,* 660–667. http://dx.doi.org/10.1191/0269215504cr746oa

Demeurisse, G., Demol, O., & Robaye, E. (1980). Motor evaluation in vascular hemiplegia. *European Neurology, 19,* 382–389.

Duncan, P. W., Bode, R. K., Min Lai, S., & Perera, S. (2003). Rasch analysis of a new stroke-specific outcome scale: The Stroke Impact Scale. *Archives of Physical Medicine and Rehabilitation, 84,* 950–963. http://dx.doi.org/10.1016/S0003-9993(03)00035-2

Duncan, P. W., Lai, S. M., & Keighley, J. (2000). Defining post-stroke recovery: Implications for design and interpretation of drug trials. *Neuropharmacology, 39,* 835–841.

Duncan, P. W., Lai, S. M., Tyler, D., Perera, S., Reker, D. M., & Studenski, S. (2002). Evaluation of proxy responses to the Stroke Impact Scale. *Stroke, 33,* 2593–2599. http://dx.doi.org/10.1161/01.STR.0000034395.06874.3E

Duncan, P. W., Reker, D. M., Horner, R. D., Samsa, G. P., Hoenig, H., LaClair, B. J., & Dudley, T. K. (2002). Performance of a mail-administered version of a stroke-specific outcome measure, the Stroke Impact Scale. *Clinical Rehabilitation, 16,* 493–505. http://dx.doi.org/10.1191/0269215502cr510oa

Duncan, P. W., Wallace, D., Lai, S. M., Johnson, D., Embretson, S., & Laster, L. J. (1999). The Stroke Impact Scale version 2.0. Evaluation of reliability, validity, and sensitivity to change. *Stroke, 30,* 2131–2140.

Duncan, P. W., Wallace, D., Studenski, S., Lai, S. M., & Johnson, D. (2001). Conceptualization of a new stroke-specific outcome measure: The Stroke Impact Scale. *Topics in Stroke Rehabilitation, 8,* 19–33. http://dx.doi.org/10.1310/BRHX-PKTA-0TUJ-UYWT

Duncan, P. W., Zorowitz, R., Bates, B., Choi, J. Y., Glasberg, J. J., Graham, G. D., . . . Reker, D. (2005). Management of adult stroke rehabilitation care: A clinical practice guideline. *Stroke, 36,* e100–e143. http://dx.doi.org/10.1161/01STR.0000180861.54180.FF

Eyssen, I. C., Steultjens, M. P., Oud, T. A., Bolt, E. M., Maasdam, A., & Dekker, J. (2011). Responsiveness of the Canadian Occupational Performance Measure. *Journal of Rehabilitation Research and Development, 48,* 517–528. http://dx.doi.org/10.1682/JRRD.2010.06.0110

Fearon, P., & Langhorne, P. (2012). Services for reducing duration of hospital care for acute stroke patients. *Cochrane Database of Systematic Reviews, 2012*(9), CD000443. http://dx.doi.org/10.1002/14651858.CD000443.pub2

Ghahramani, Z., & Wolpert, D. M. (1997). Modular decomposition in visuomotor learning. *Nature, 386,* 392–395.

Goodbody, S. J., & Wolpert, D. M. (1998). Temporal and amplitude generalization in motor learning. *Journal of Neurophysiology, 79,* 1825–1838.

Heilman, K. M., Rothi, L. J., & Valenstein, E. (1982). Two forms of ideomotor apraxia. *Neurology, 32,* 342–346. http://dx.doi.org/10.1212/WNL.32.4.342

Heller, A., Wade, D. T., Wood, V. A., Sunderland, A., Hewer, R. L., & Ward, E. (1987). Arm function after stroke: Measurement and recovery over the first three months. *Journal of Neurology, Neurosurgery and Psychiatry, 50,* 714–719. http://dx.doi.org/10.1136/jnnp.50.6.714

Hlustik, P., & Mayer, M. (2006). Paretic hand in stroke: From motor cortical plasticity research to rehabilitation. *Cognitive and Behavioral Neurology, 19,* 34–40. http://dx.doi.org/10.1097/00146965-200603000-00004

Hubbard, I. J., Parsons, M. W., Neilson, C., & Carey, L. M. (2009). Task-specific training: Evidence for and translation to clinical practice. *Occupational Therapy International, 16,* 175–189. http://dx.doi.org/10.1002/oti.275

Jebsen, R. H., Taylor, N., Trieschmann, R. B., Trotter, M. J., & Howard, L. A. (1969). An objective and standardized test of hand function. *Archives of Physical Medicine and Rehabilitation, 50,* 311–319.

Jorgensen, H. S., Nakayama, H., Raaschou, H. O., Vive-Larsen, J., Stoier, M., & Olsen, T. S. (1995). Outcome and time course of recovery in stroke. Part II: Time course of recovery. The Copenhagen Stroke Study. *Archives of Physical Medicine and Rehabilitation, 76,* 406–412.

Karni, A., Meyer, G., Jezzard, P., Adams, M. M., Turner, R., & Ungerleider, L. G. (1995). Functional MRI evidence for adult motor cortex plasticity during motor skill learning. *Nature, 377,* 155–158.

Karni, A., Meyer, G., Rey-Hipolito, C., Jezzard, P., Adams, M. M., Turner, R., & Ungerleider, L. G. (1998). The acquisition of skilled motor performance: Fast and slow experience-driven changes in primary motor cortex. *Proceedings of the National Academy of Sciences, USA, 95,* 861–868.

Kleim, J. A., Barbay, S., & Nudo, R. J. (1998). Functional reorganization of the rat motor cortex following motor skill learning. *Journal of Neurophysiology, 80,* 3321–3325.

Kleim, J. A., & Jones, T. A. (2008). Principles of experience-dependent neural plasticity: Implications for rehabilitation after brain damage. *Journal of Speech, Language, and Hearing Research, 51,* S225–S239. http://dx.doi.org/10.1044/1092-4388(2008/018)

Kleim, J. A., Jones, T. A., & Schallert, T. (2003). Motor enrichment and the induction of plasticity before or after brain injury. *Neurochemical Research, 28,* 1757–1769.

Knutson, J. S., Harley, M. Y., Hisel, T. Z., Hogan, S. D., Maloney, M. M., & Chae, J. (2012). Contralaterally controlled functional electrical stimulation for upper extremity hemiplegia: An early-phase randomized clinical trial in subacute stroke patients. *Neurorehabilitation and Neural Repair, 26,* 239–246. http://dx.doi.org/10.1177/1545968311419301

Krakauer, J. W. (2006). Motor learning: Its relevance to stroke recovery and neurorehabilitation. *Current Opinion in Neurology, 19*(1), 84–90.

Kwakkel, G., Kollen, B., & Lindeman, E. (2004). Understanding the pattern of functional recovery after stroke: Facts and theories. *Restorative Neurology and Neuroscience, 22,* 281–299.

Kwakkel, G., Kollen, B. J., van der Grond, J., & Prevo, A. J. (2003). Probability of regaining dexterity in the flaccid upper limb: Impact of severity of paresis and time since onset in acute stroke. *Stroke, 34,* 2181–2186. http://dx.doi.org/10.1080/09638280802061878

Lang, C. E. (2012). Impaired motor control. In A. Guccione, R. Wong, & D. Avers (Eds.), *Geriatric physical therapy* (pp. 272–291). New York: Elsevier.

Lang, C. E., & Beebe, J. A. (2007). Relating movement control at 9 upper extremity segments to loss of hand function in people with chronic hemiparesis. *Neurorehabilitation and Neural Repair, 21,* 279–291. http://dx.doi.org/10.1177/1545968306296964

Lang, C. E., Bland, M. D., Bailey, R. R., Schaefer, S. Y., & Birkenmeier, R. L. (2013). Assessment of upper extremity impairment, function, and activity after stroke: Foundations for clinical decision making. *Journal of Hand Therapy, 26,* 104–115. http://dx.doi.org/10.1016/j.jht.2012.06.005

Lang, C. E., Macdonald, J. R., Reisman, D. S., Boyd, L., Jacobson Kimberley, T., Schindler-Ivens, S. M., . . . Scheets, P. L. (2009). Observation of amounts of movement practice provided during stroke rehabilitation. *Archives of Physical Medicine and Rehabilitation, 90,* 1692–1968. http://dx.doi.org/10.1016/j.apmr.2009.04.005

Law, M., Baptiste, S., McColl, M., Opzoomer, A., Polatajko, H., & Pollock, N. (1990). The Canadian Occupational Performance Measure: An outcome measure for occupational therapy. *Canadian Journal of Occupational Therapy, 57,* 82–87. http://dx.doi.org/10.1177/000841749005700207

Lazar, R. M., Minzer, B., Antoniello, D., Festa, J. R., Krakauer, J. W., & Marshall, R. S. (2010). Improvement in aphasia scores after stroke is well predicted by initial severity. *Stroke, 41,* 1485–1488. http://dx.doi.org/10.1161/STROKEAHA.109.577338

Leach, E., Cornwell, P., Fleming, J., & Haines, T. (2010). Patient centered goal-setting in a subacute rehabilitation setting. *Disability and Rehabilitation, 32,* 159–172. http://dx.doi.org/10.3109/09638280903036605

Liepert, J., Graef, S., Uhde, I., Leidner, O., & Weiller, C. (2000). Training-induced changes of motor cortex representations in stroke patients. *Acta Neurologica Scandinavica, 101,* 321–326. http://dx.doi.org/10.1034/j.1600-0404.2000.90337a.x

Lindgren, I., Jonsson, A. C., Norrving, B., & Lindgren, A. (2007). Shoulder pain after stroke: A prospective population-based study. *Stroke, 38,* 343–348. http://dx.doi.org/10.1161/01.STR.0000254598.16739.4e

Lyle, R. C. (1981). A performance test for assessment of upper limb function in physical rehabilitation treatment and research. *International Journal of Rehabilitation Research, 4,* 483–492.

Mathiowetz, V., Kashman, N., Volland, G., Weber, K., Dowe, M., & Rogers, S. (1985). Grip and pinch strength: Normative data for adults. *Archives of Physical Medicine and Rehabilitation, 66,* 69–74.

Mathiowetz, V., Volland, G., Kashman, N., & Weber, K. (1985). Adult norms for the Box and Block Test of manual dexterity. *American Journal of Occupational Therapy, 39,* 386–391. http://dx.doi.org/10.5014/ajot.39.6.386

Mathiowetz, V., Weber, K., Kashman, N., & Volland, G. (1985). Adult norms for the Nine Hole Peg Test of finger dexterity. *OTJR: Occupation, Participation and Health, 5,* 24–38.

Mathiowetz, V., Weber, K., Volland, G., & Kashman, N. (1984). Reliability and validity of grip and pinch strength evaluations. *Journal of Hand Surgery, 9,* 222–226. http://dx.doi.org/10.1016/S0363-5023(84)80146-X

Morton, S. M., & Bastian, A. J. (2009). Can rehabilitation help ataxia? *Neurology, 73,* 1818–1819. http://dx.doi.org/10.1212/WNL.0b013e3181c33b21

Nijland, R. H., van Wegen, E. E., Harmeling-van der Wel, B. C., & Kwakkel, G. (2010). Presence of finger extension and shoulder abduction within 72 hours after stroke predicts functional recovery: Early prediction of functional outcome after stroke: The EPOS cohort study. *Stroke, 41,* 745–750. http://dx.doi.org/10.1161/STROKEAHA.109.572065

Nudo, R. J. (2006). Mechanisms for recovery of motor function following cortical damage. *Current Opinions in Neurobiology, 16,* 638–644. http://dx.doi.org/10.1016/j.conb.2006.10.004

Nudo, R. J. (2007). Postinfarct cortical plasticity and behavioral recovery. *Stroke, 38,* 840–845. http://dx.doi.org/10.1161/01.STR.0000247943.12887.d2

Nudo, R. J., & Milliken, G. W. (1996). Reorganization of movement representations in primary motor cortex following focal ischemic infarcts in adult squirrel monkeys. *Journal of Neurophysiology, 75,* 2144–2149.

Nudo, R. J., Milliken, G. W., Jenkins, W. M., & Merzenich, M. M. (1996). Use-dependent alterations of movement representations in primary motor cortex of adult squirrel monkeys. *Journal of Neuroscience, 16,* 785–807.

Nudo, R. J., Plautz, E. J., & Frost, S. B. (2001). Role of adaptive plasticity in recovery of function after damage to motor cortex. *Muscle and Nerve, 24,* 1000–1019.

Pascual-Leone, A., Grafman, J., & Hallett, M. (1994). Modulation of cortical motor output maps during development of implicit and explicit knowledge. *Science, 263,* 1287–1289.

Peterson, G. B. (2004). A day of great illumination: B. F. Skinner's discovery of shaping. *Journal of the Experi-*

mental *Analysis of Behavior, 82*, 317–328. http://dx.doi.org/10.1901/jeab.2004.82-317

Petreska, B., Adriani, M., Blanke, O., & Billard, A. G. (2007). Apraxia: A review. *Progress in Brain Research, 164*, 61–83.

Plautz, E. J., Milliken, G. W., & Nudo, R. J. (2000). Effects of repetitive motor training on movement representations in adult squirrel monkeys: Role of use versus learning. *Neurobiology of Learning and Memory, 74*, 27–55. http://dx.doi.org/10.1006/nlme.1999.3934

Prabhakaran, S., Zarahn, E., Riley, C., Speizer, A., Chong, J. Y., Lazar, R. M., . . . Krakauer, J. W. (2008). Inter-individual variability in the capacity for motor recovery after ischemic stroke. *Neurorehabilitation and Neural Repair, 22*, 64–71. http://dx.doi.org/10.1177/1545968307305302

Prager, E. M., & Lang, C. E. (2012). Predictive ability of 2-day measurement of active range of motion on 3-mo upper extremity motor function in people with post-stroke hemiparesis. *American Journal of Occupational Therapy, 66*, 35–41. http://dx.doi.org/10.5014/ajot.2012.002683

Rebeiro, K. L., & Polgar, J. M. (1999). Enabling occupational performance: Optimal experiences in therapy. *Canadian Journal of Occupational Therapy, 66*, 14–22. http://dx.doi.org/10.1177/000841749906600102

Roy, C. W., Sands, M. R., & Hill, L. D. (1994). Shoulder pain in acutely admitted hemiplegics. *Clinical Rehabilitation, 8*, 334–340. http://dx.doi.org/10.1177/026921559400800410

Roy, C. W., Sands, M. R., Hill, L. D., Harrison, A., & Marshall, S. (1995). The effect of shoulder pain on outcome of acute hemiplegia. *Clinical Rehabilitation, 9*, 21–27. http://dx.doi.org/10.1177/026921559500900103

Sathian, K., Buxbaum, L. J., Cohen, L. G., Krakauer, J. W., Lang, C. E., Corbetta, M., & Fitzpatrick, S. M. (2011). Neurological principles and rehabilitation of action disorders: Common clinical deficits. *Neurorehabilitation and Neural Repair, 25*, 21S–32S. http://dx.doi.org/10.1177/1545968311410941

Schaefer, S. Y., & Lang, C. E. (2012). Using dual tasks to test immediate transfer of training between naturalistic movements: A proof-of-principle study. *Journal of Motor Behavior, 44*, 313–327. http://dx.doi.org/10.1080/00222895.2012.708367

Schaefer, S. Y., Patterson, C. B., & Lang, C. E. (2013). Transfer of training between distinct motor tasks after stroke: Implications for task-specific approaches to upper-extremity neurorehabilitation. *Neuroreha-

bilitation and Neural Repair, 27*, 602–612. http://dx.doi.org/10.1177/1545968313481279

Shadmehr, R., & Moussavi, Z. M. (2000). Spatial generalization from learning dynamics of reaching movements. *Journal of Neuroscience, 20*, 7807–7815.

Shepherd, R. B. (2001). Exercise and training to optimize functional motor performance in stroke: Driving neural reorganization? *Neural Plasticity, 8*, 121–129. http://dx.doi.org/10.1155/NP.2001.121

Simek, E. M., McPhate, L., & Haines, T. P. (2012). Adherence to and efficacy of home exercise programs to prevent falls: A systematic review and meta-analysis of the impact of exercise program characteristics. *Preventive Medicine, 55*, 262–275. http://dx.doi.org/10.1016/j.ypmed.2012.07.007

Spink, M. J., Fotoohabadi, M. R., Wee, E., Landorf, K. B., Hill, K. D., Lord, S. R., & Menz, H. B. (2011). Predictors of adherence to a multifaceted podiatry intervention for the prevention of falls in older people. *BMC Geriatrics, 11*, 51. http://dx.doi.org/10.1186/1471-2318-11-51

Stinear, C. M., Barber, P. A., Coxon, J. P., Fleming, M. K., & Byblow, W. D. (2008). Priming the motor system enhances the effects of upper limb therapy in chronic stroke. *Brain, 131*, 1381–1390. http://dx.doi.org/10.1093/brain/awn051

Sunderland, A., Tinson, D., Bradley, L., & Hewer, R. L. (1989). Arm function after stroke. An evaluation of grip strength as a measure of recovery and a prognostic indicator. *Journal of Neurology, Neurosurgery and Psychiatry, 52*, 1267–1272.

Taub, E., Miller, N. E., Novack, T. A., Cook, E. W., 3rd, Fleming, W. C., Nepomuceno, C. S., . . . Crago, J. E. (1993). Technique to improve chronic motor deficit after stroke. *Archives of Physical Medicine and Rehabilitation, 74*, 347–354.

Taub, E., Uswatte, G., Mark, V. W., Morris, D. M., Barman, J., Bowman, M. H., . . . Bishop-McKay, S. (2013). Method for enhancing real-world use of a more affected arm in chronic stroke: Transfer package of constraint-induced movement therapy. *Stroke, 44*, 1383–1388. http://dx.doi.org/10.1161/STROKEAHA.111.000559

Taub, E., Uswatte, G., & Pidikiti, R. (1999). Constraint-induced movement therapy: A new family of techniques with broad application to physical rehabilitation—A clinical review. *Journal of Rehabilitation Research and Development, 36*, 237–251.

Teasell, R., Foley, N., Salter, K., Boghal, S., Jutai, J., & Speechley, M. (2008). *Evidence-based review of stroke rehabilitation.* London, Ontario: University of Western Ontario.

Turner-Stokes, L., & Jackson, D. (2002). Shoulder pain after stroke: A review of the evidence base to inform the development of an integrated care pathway. *Clinical Rehabilitation, 16,* 276–298. http://dx.doi.org/10.1191/0269215502cr491oa

U.S. Department of Defense, & U.S. Department of Veterans Affairs. (2010). *VA/DoD clinical practice guidelines for the management of stroke rehabilitation.* Washington, DC: Author.

Uswatte, G., Taub, E., Morris, D., Light, K., & Thompson, P. A. (2006). The Motor Activity Log–28: Assessing daily use of the hemiparetic arm after stroke. *Neurology, 67,* 1189–1194. http://dx.doi.org/10.1212/01.wnl.0000238164.90657.c2

Uswatte, G., Taub, E., Morris, D., Vignolo, M., & McCulloch, K. (2005). Reliability and validity of the upper-extremity Motor Activity Log–14 for measuring real-world arm use. *Stroke, 36,* 2493–2496. http://dx.doi.org/10.1161/01.STR.0000185928.90848.2e

Wanklyn, P., Forster, A., & Young, J. (1996). Hemiplegic shoulder pain (HSP): Natural history and investigation of associated features. *Disability and Rehabilitation, 18,* 497–501.

Wheaton, L. A., & Hallett, M. (2007). Ideomotor apraxia: A review. *Journal of Neurological Science, 260,* 1–10.

Winstein, C. J., Miller, J. P., Blanton, S., Taub, E., Uswatte, G., Morris, D., . . . Wolf, S. (2003). Methods for a multisite randomized trial to investigate the effect of constraint-induced movement therapy in improving upper extremity function among adults recovering from a cerebrovascular stroke. *Neurorehabilitation and Neural Repair, 17,* 137–152.

Winstein, C. J., & Stewart, J. C. (2006). Conditions of task practice for individuals with neurologic impairments. In M. E. Selzer, S. Clarke, L. Cohen, P. Duncan, & F. H. Gage (Eds.), *Textbook of neural repair and rehabilitation* (Vol. 2, pp. 89–102). Cambridge, England: Cambridge University Press.

Woldag, H., Stupka, K., & Hummelsheim, H. (2010). Repetitive training of complex hand and arm movements with shaping is beneficial for motor improvement in patients after stroke. *Journal of Rehabilitation Medicine, 42*(6), 582–587.

Wolf, S. L., Catlin, P. A., Ellis, M., Archer, A. L., Morgan, B., & Piacentino, A. (2001). Assessing Wolf motor function test as outcome measure for research in patients after stroke. *Stroke, 32,* 1635–1639.

Wolf, S. L., Winstein, C. J., Miller, J. P., Taub, E., Uswatte, G., Morris, D., . . . Nichols-Larsen, D. (2006). Effect of constraint-induced movement therapy on upper extremity function 3 to 9 months after stroke: The EXCITE randomized clinical trial. *JAMA, 296,* 2095–2104. http://dx.doi.org/10.1001/jama.296.17.2095

Yozbatiran, N., Der-Yeghiaian, L., & Cramer, S. C. (2008). A standardized approach to performing the action research arm test. *Neurorehabilitation and Neural Repair, 22,* 78–90. http://dx.doi.org/10.1177/1545968307305353

Yuen, H. K., Wang, E., Holthaus, K., Vogtle, L. K., Sword, D., Breland, H. L., & Kamen, D. L. (2013). Self-reported versus objectively assessed exercise adherence. *American Journal of Occupational Therapy, 67,* 484–489. http://dx.doi.org/10.5014/ajot.2013.007575

Zarahn, E., Alon, L., Ryan, S. L., Lazar, R. M., Vry, M. S., Weiller, C., . . . Krakauer, J. W. (2011). Prediction of motor recovery using initial impairment and fMRI 48 h poststroke. *Cerebral Cortex, 21,* 2712–2721. http://dx.doi.org/10.1093/cercor/bhr047

Subject Index

Note. Page numbers in *italic* refer to exhibits, figures, and tables.

dusting table, 93
DVD, placing into DVD player, 122

E
eating soup, 39
emptying trash can, 97
e-reader, navigating, 60
eyeglasses, donning and doffing, 50

F
face, shaving, 52
fastening clothes to clothesline, 86
fastening paperclip to papers, 77
fastening twist tie to bread bag, 113
feedback, value of, 22
filing fingernails, 45
filling out forms, 78
fine motor control, decreased
    defined, 30
    leisure tasks for, 118, 119, 123, 125, 126, 130
    productivity tasks for, 55, 56, 57, 58, 60, 61, 73, 75, 77, 78, 80, 83, 86, 89, 90, 113
    self-care tasks for, 32, 34, 42, 43, 54
fingernails
    clipping, 32
    filing, 45
fishing line, casting, 117
flipping light switch, 62
floor, sweeping, 69
flowers, planting, 128
foil, wrapping food in, 103
folding socks, 37
folding towels, 66
food, cutting, 63
forms, filling out, 78
fractionated movement, loss of, 8

G
gloves, donning and doffing, 54
goals
    matching with specific tasks, 15, 16, 17, 18, 19
    setting, 12–13
    for UE function, 17, 18, 19
golfing, 129
grading tasks, changing, 19–21, 20, 21
grasping paper towel from roll, 99
grasping shoes from shoebox, 44
grip strength, decreased
    defined, 30
    leisure tasks for, 117–118, 129
    productivity tasks for, 59, 63–69, 71–74, 76, 79, 81, 84, 87–88, 90–91, 93, 95–96, 98–101, 103, 105–110, 112, 114–116
    self-care tasks for, 33, 35, 37–41, 44, 46, 50–51
grocery bag, tying, 90

H
hair
    brushing, 35
    washing, 49
handwriting, 56

hanging clothes on hangers, 67
headphones, donning, 100
hemispatial neglect, 135–136
home exercise programs, 137–141, 138, 139, 141
hypertonicity, 8
hypotonicity, 8

J
jacket
    donning and doffing, 40
    zipping, 36

L
laundry, stacking, 94
laundry basket, removing towels from, 65
leaves, raking, 115
leisure tasks
    bowling, 121
    casting fishing line, 117
    golfing, 129
    lighting candle, 130
    placing DVD into DVD player, 122
    planting flowers, 128
    playing bingo, 126
    playing cards, 120
    playing Connect Four, 124
    rolling dice, 119
    scrapbooking, 118
    swinging tennis racquet, 127
    taking a photo, 131
    threading beads onto necklace, 125
    turning pages of book, 123
letter, mailing, 112
lids, removing, 64
light switch, flipping, 62
lighting candle, 130
locking door, 79
long-term potentiation (LTP), 2

M
mailing a letter, 112
MAL (Motor Activity Log), 12
MI (Motricity Index), 15
microwave, setting, 104
money, counting, 58
Motor Activity Log (MAL), 12
motor capabilities, challenging, 15–19
Motricity Index (MI), 15
mouse, clicking, 57

N
navigating digital tablet or e-reader, 60
neglect, 7
neurogenesis, 2
nut and bolt, assembling, 75

O
opening and closing umbrella, 47
opening containers, 87
opening door, 70

Citation Index

Note. Page numbers in *italic* refer to exhibits, figures, and tables.

Fleming, M. K., 2
Fleming, W. C., 2
Foley, N., 2
Forster, A., 134
Fotoohabadi, M. R., 140
Frost, S. B., 2
Fucetola, R., 9

G
Ghahramani, Z., 3
Glasberg, J. J., 9, 12
Goodbody, S. J., 3
Gowland, C. K., 12
Graef, S., 2
Grafman, J., 2
Graham, G. D., 9, 12
Griffiths, J., 12

H
Haines, T., 12, 137
Haines, T. P., 140
Hallett, M., 2, 7, 135
Harley, M. Y., 2
Harmeling-van der Wel, B. C., 13
Harris, H., 9
Harrison, A., 134
Heilman, K. M., 135
Heller, A., *10*
Hewer, R. L., *10*
Hill, K. D., 140
Hill, L. D., 134
Hisel, T. Z., 2
Hlustik, P., 2
Hoenig, H., 12
Hogan, S. D., 2
Holthaus, K., 140
Horner, R. D., 12
Howard, L. A., 12
Hubbard, I. J., 1, 2, 3
Huijbregts, M., 12

J
Jackson, D., 134
Jacobson Kimberley, T., 140
Jebsen, R. H., 12
Jenkins, W. M., 2
Jezzard, P., 2
Johnson, D., 12
Jones, T. A., 2, 3, 137
Jonsson, A. C., 134
Jorgensen, H. S., 13
Jutai, J., 2

K
Kamen, D. L., 140
Karlsson, G. M., 135
Karni, A., 2
Kashman, N., 9, *10*, 12
Keighley, J., 13

Kimberley, T. J., 2
Kincade, M. J., 7, 135
Kleim, J. A., 2, 3, 137
Knutson, J. S., 2
Kollen, B., 13
Kollen, B. J., 13
Krakauer, J. W., 7, 8, 13, 134, 135
Kwakkel, G., 13

L
LaClair, B. J., 12
Ladavas, E., 7, 135
Lai, S. M., 12, 13
Lambert, C. L., 12
Landorf, K. B., 140
Lang, C. E., 3, 7, 8, 9, 13, 27, 133, 134, 135, 140
Lang, C.E., 16, 134
Langhorne, P., 137
Laster, L. J., 12
Law, M., 12, 15
Lazar, R. M., 13
Leach, E., 12, 137
Legg, L. A., 137
Leidner, O., 2
Lewis, C., 7, 135
Lewis, S. M., 2
Liepert, J., 2
Light, K., 12
Lindeman, E., 13
Lindgren, A., 134
Lindgren, I., 134
Lord, S. R., 140
Lyle, R. C., 9, 17

M
Maasdam, A., 12
Macdonald, J. R., 140
Maloney, M. M., 2
Mark, V. W., 2
Marshall, R. S., 13
Marshall, S., 134
Masters, L., 12
Masters, L. M., 12
Mathiowetz, V., 9, *10*, 12
Mayer, M., 2
McBay, C., 12
McColl, M., 12, 15
McCulloch, K., 12
McPhate, L., 140
Menz, H. B., 140
Merzenich, M. M., 2
Meyer, G., 2
Miller, J. P., 2
Miller, N. E., 2
Milliken, G. W., 2
Min Lai, S., 12
Minzer, B., 13
Morgan, B., 12
Morris, D. M., 2, 12